THE DASH DIET

Keeping your heart alive, one meal at a time

Summary to the DASH Diet

According to a number of reports from credible sources, there are many medical conditions that we suffer from as a result of the lifestyle choices that we make. One of the most common causes of such conditions is the food that we eat. It is important to make sure that we watch what we eat. Your body will be harmed if you don't watch for what you need to do.

The DASH Diet is one of the most popular diets to use today. As a matter of fact, it is recommended over the typical American diet and is touted as one of the best diets ever. This can be utilized to prevent hypertension and other possible life-threatening conditions that might result from not watching your diet carefully.

Based on a recent survey, three diets were selected as the best diets of the year. The DASH Diet was awarded the top spot in a study followed by the TLC and Weight Watchers diets in that order of preference.

It is important to take note that this diet is not designed to help you cut lose some pounds, but if you do so in the process, then good for you. The main aim of the DASH Diet is to prevent the threat of blood pressure. As a matter of fact, the DASH Diet is not even referred to as a diet by the federal government that proposed the study and further recommended the conclusions, but it is referred to as an eating plan.

In the event that you have come across other diets like the TLC diet, the Mediterranean Diet, the Vegetarian diet or even the Mayo Clinic Diet, it should be easier for you to work with the DASH Diet. The pretext to the DASH Diet is based on the fact that it is a lot easier to fight blood pressure by making sure that you eat healthy. Did you know that when you are on this diet you will also be able to keep a good waistline? Well, how about that!

The DASH diet simply works on the advantages that you will get from the intake of mineral foods. These include things like potassium, protein and calcium. These usually go a long way in ensuring that you can prevent high blood pressure. You do not need to spend a lot of time monitoring the amount of each that you take in, but all you have to do is to make sure that your diet has fruits and vegetables and you will be good to go. Apart from that, the most important thing that you need to do is to cut down on your salt intake.

Selecting the DASH Diet Plan For You

Before you set out on the diet, you should first of all make sure that you have an idea of how much food you want to eat as far as calories are concerned. The amount of calories that you need will depend on your activity level and your age group. With these in mind, you should be able to select the best diet plan for your goals.

High Blood Pressure

The report also takes a look at blood pressure and gives you some basics that you need to know to combat blood pressure and related issues. Do you know what the recommended blood pressure for optimal body performance is? You have to take note of your body's system and be keen on the changes to your body.

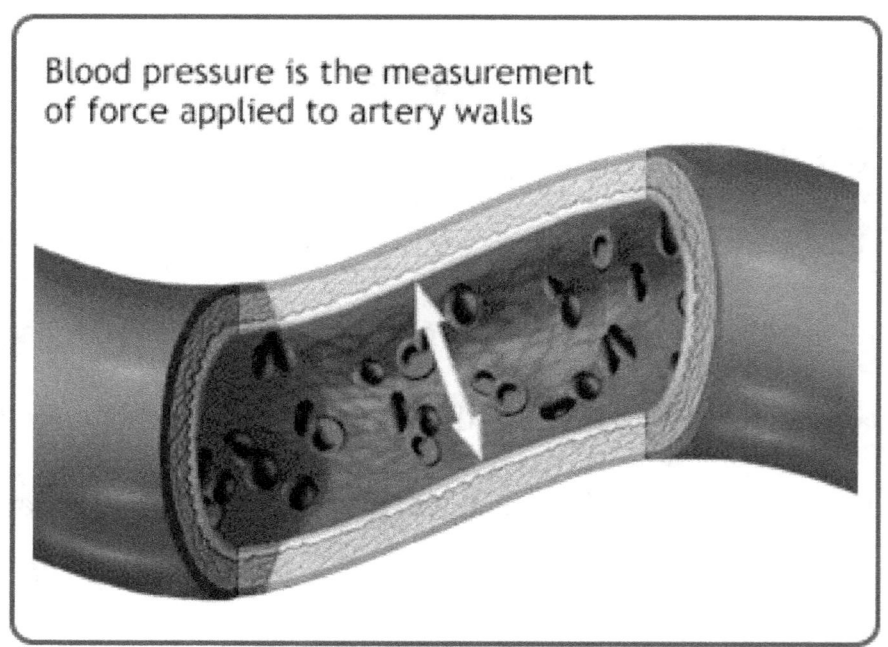

The measure of blood pressure is important to your body's overall health but you particularly have to be certain about how your body will respond. You need to know that in most cases there are no symptoms for high blood pressure, and on the same note a lot of people are usually caught off guard if they develop complications from it. Their artery walls can progressively wear out without anyone noticing or even feeling a thing as it happens. Therefore, the only way through which you can be able to get ahead of this situation is to track your blood pressure and to eat a very good diet.

There are a number of eating plans that are discussed in this report that you can make use of in a bid to get the best diet plan running. You'll also learn about the right foods for you to buy for your diet as well as what must be avoided at all times. In this list, there are many foods that you can use in the DASH Diet as well as a number of substitutes.

Many of the important things tackled in this book include some of the most commonly asked questions with regards to the DASH Diet. This attempts to answer all the questions and concerns that you might have with regards to the diet and tries to give you peace of mind when you set out on the diet plan.

Finally, there are some recipes in this book that you can use for at least a week when starting out on the diet. These recipes are very easy to prepare, and should take as short a time as you can imagine. The instructions are precise and easy to follow. The best thing about this is that the meals also have their different food contents weighed appropriately and indicated so you'll know how much of what you are taking in.

The most important thing about this book is that you'll get an insight into the DASH Diet. You have a lot of alternatives in front of you, and with the DASH diet, you will take a huge step towards protecting your heart and your life. It's a critical part of your health that must work well if things are to be safe.

Contents

Abstract

We live in a world where so many things are drastically changing, and over time we must either adapt our lifestyles or learn to work with new ones. This is of course in terms of the dietary needs and plans that we keep in our daily lives.

There are several life threatening conditions and illnesses that come up as a result of the dietary lifestyles that we lead, and because of this it is important that we take precautions and watch what we eat. One of the best ways to beat this kind of change is to practice a healthy diet. There are so many of these that have since been introduced in the world, and one of the most important of them all is the DASH Diet.

An organ of the National Institute of Health in the US came up with the Dietary Approaches to Stop Hypertension (DASH) diet in a bid to fight the increasing spread of hypertension and other related conditions.

Basically, this diet is designed around fruits, whole grains, vegetables and low-fat dairy foods. Some of these foods include poultry, fish, meat, and beans. However, there is also the inclusion of some sweetened foods like beverages, added fats or even red meat. This diet is aimed at controlling hypertension and encouraging a healthy lifestyle to prevent it in the future. The USDA strongly recommends this plan based on the research and results relating to this diet.

Introduction

Did you know that you have a higher chance of developing high blood pressure as a result of your diet? According to recent studies, a lot of people are suffering today from lifestyle-induced medical conditions. This is primarily as a result of the diets that we keep. Some of the foods that we eat from time to time can cause hypertension to develop.

Hypertension, or high blood pressure, is usually induced by taking in foods that are rich in sodium (common salt). The first step towards preventing hypertension would is to cut down on your salt intake. You'll also need to practice the DASH Diet for the best results.

The DASH Diet could help you do more than just lower your salt intake. It will also promote the development of a healthy lifestyle so you can lose weight and control this condition before it could be worse.

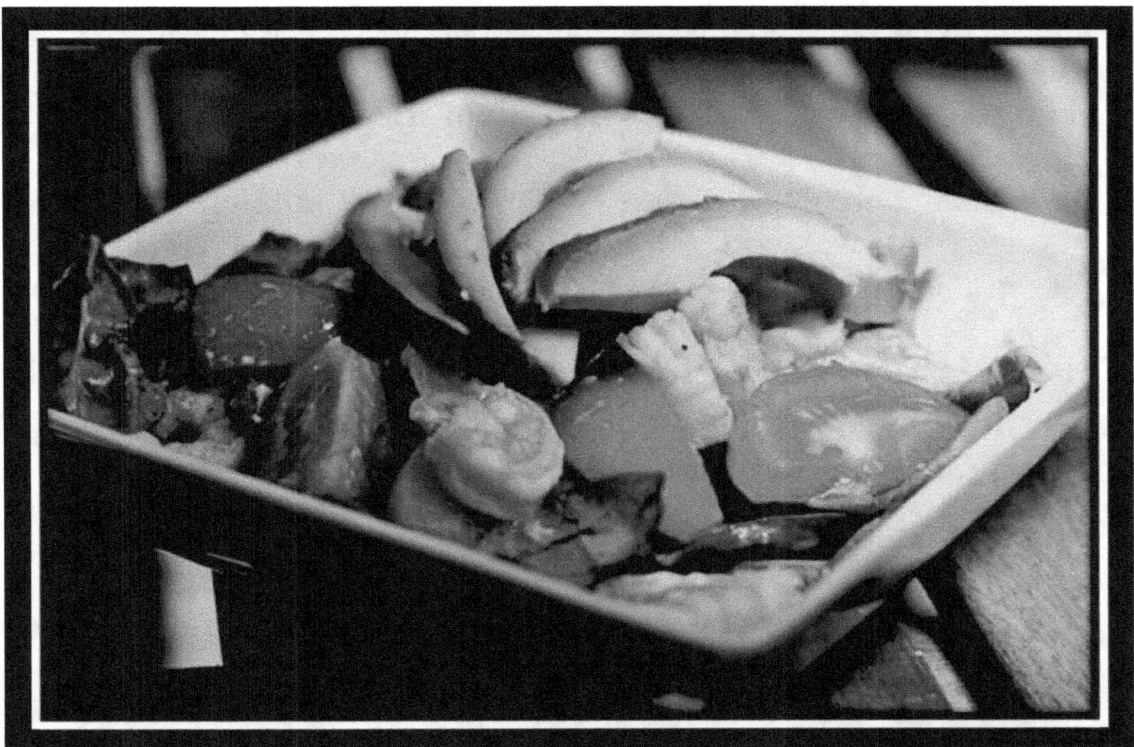

Through this report, you'll get the information you can use to get on the path to the DASH Diet in the event that you are not already on one or you are considering one already. It is a great plan for beginners and novices alike.

Apart from that, you will also come across a number of menus and useful recipes that you can use when you are planning to live off of the DASH Diet. According to the National High Blood Pressure Education Program, your body only requires 2300 mg of sodium each day. This is also considered the recommended amount by the US Dietary Guidelines for Americans and many other respectable authorities all around the world. Naturally, if you can keep your intake of sodium to 1500 mg a day, you should make an important step towards fighting hypertension.

Relevant studies have recently indicated that your blood pressure can decline when you reduce your total daily sodium intake. Normal DASH menus usually contain 2300 mg of sodium to help you lower your blood pressure. However, you should try and keep this to 1500 mg per day for the best results. This is also in stark comparison to what most people consume on a daily basis.

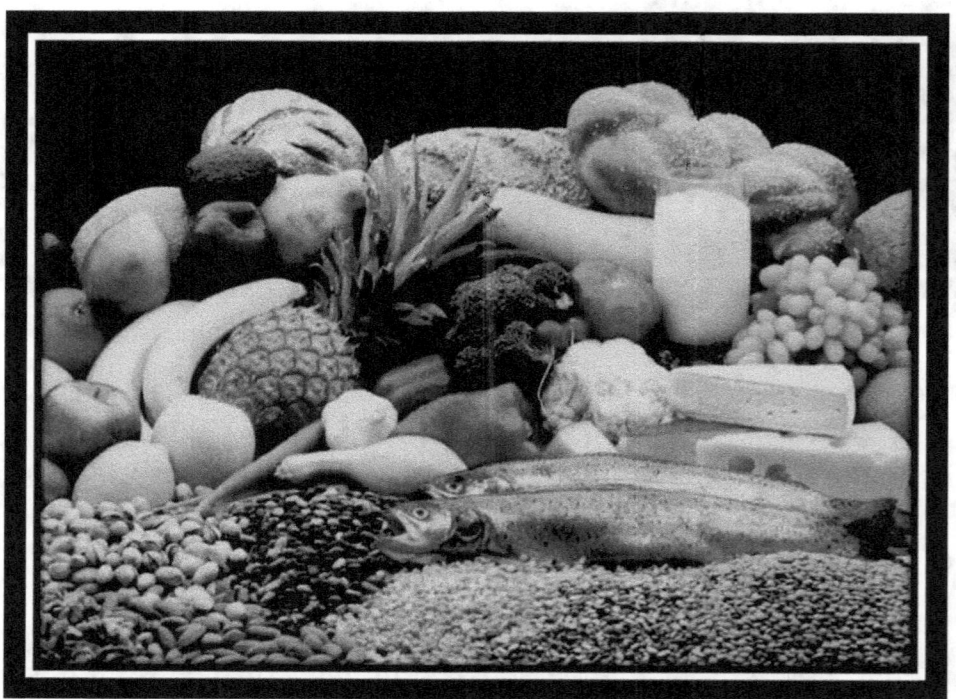

In as much as the relevant authorities recommend anything lower that 2300 mg per day, it is important to take note that on a daily basis, most adults usually take more than 3000 mg per day. Men often use 4200 mg each day while women use 3300 mg in their diets.

The dangers are as real as the statistics, and this is why there are so many people in the world who suffer from high blood pressure. These include people who are not fully aware of how they are suffering from this condition. With respect to this, high blood pressure has become one of the most common ailments that people go to hospitals for but anyone can take the path to becoming safe from this condition by simply practicing a good diet.

High Blood Pressure

Before we look into the DASH diet and what it is all about, its benefits and so forth, it is important that we understand what high blood pressure is all about. Blood pressure refers to the natural force of blood as it passes through artery walls. Blood pressure is usually measured in millimeters of mercury (Hg). It is denoted with two different numbers, the diastolic pressure and the systolic pressure.

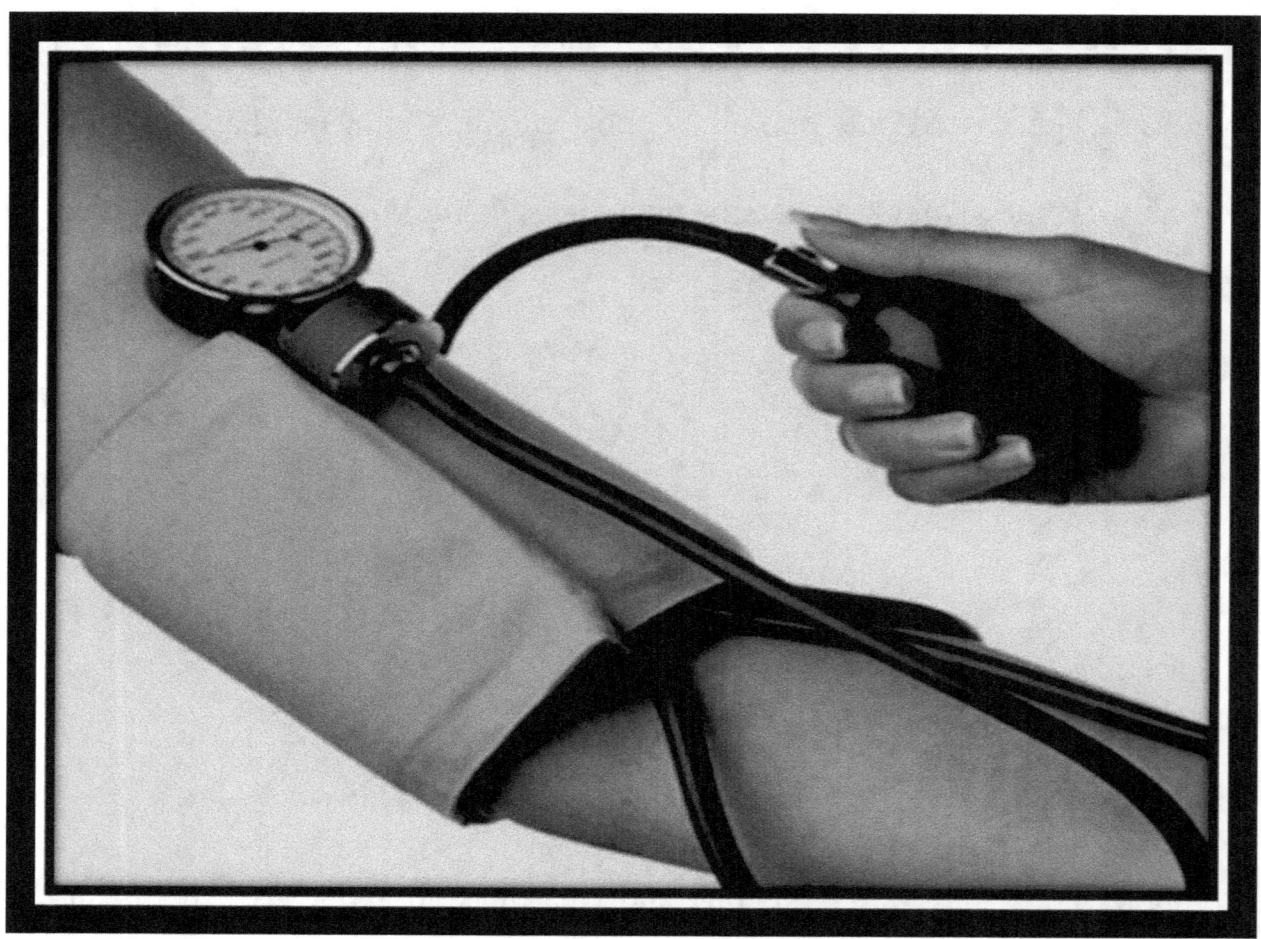

Diastolic pressure refers to that point where the heart relaxes in between beats, while systolic pressure refers to the point where the heart beats.

It is important to note that your blood pressure can rise or fall throughout the day due to your diet or the environment you are exposed to. Your heart will naturally beat faster when you are exposed to some danger or when you are threatened in any way. Anything that might surprise you might also cause your heart to beat faster. However when you are calm relaxed or composed, your heart will ease up.

When you have high blood pressure, your heart will beat faster and will keep on doing this for a long time. This is very dangerous to your health because your heart will be in overdrive. Your heart is forced to work harder and faster than its normal working conditions. In such a situation, the high force of the blood can be a danger to the arteries and other organs including the heart, your eyes, the kidney and brain.

You have to be on top of your blood pressure at all times because high blood pressure rarely has any symptoms or warning signs that can alert you to seek medical help. In most cases the impact is sporadic and unexpected. Once it develops in your body and is unchecked, it will last as long as you are alive. In the event that this is not monitored, you will be risking blindness, stroke, heart and kidney disease plus other conditions that might come about because of your blood pressure.

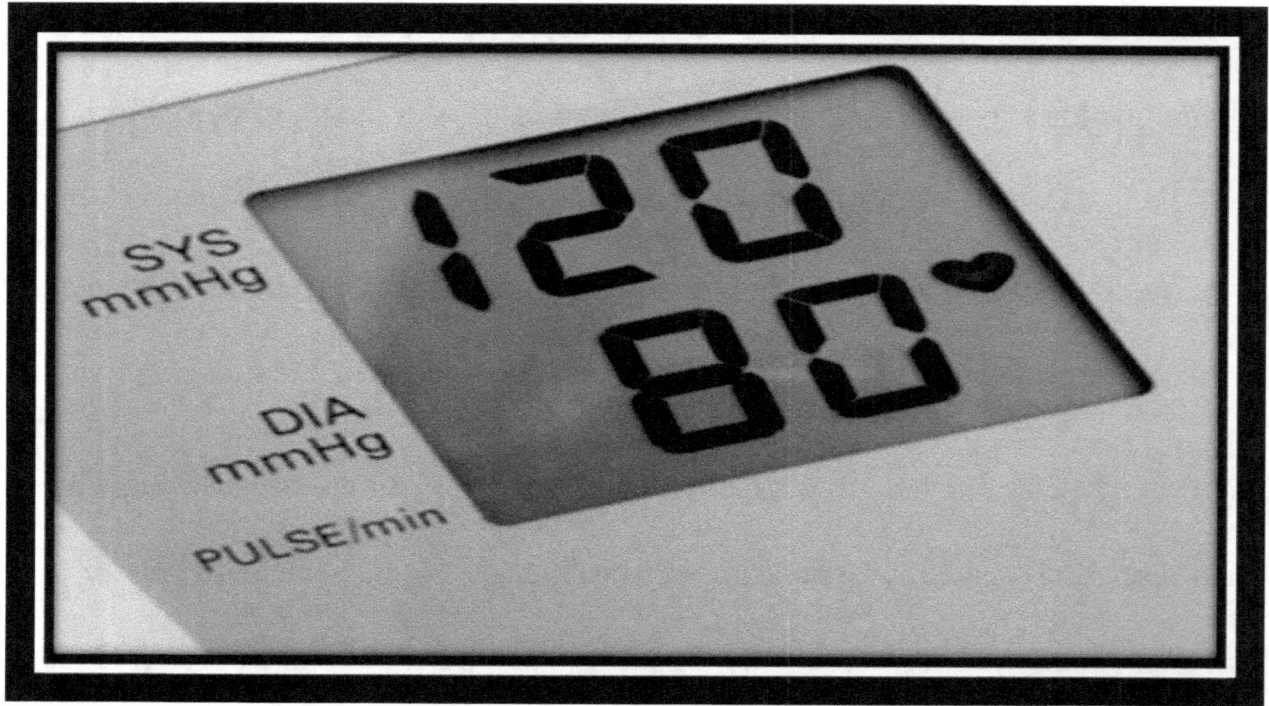

Statistics indicate that more than 70 million people in the United States suffer from high blood pressure. That's at least one in every three people in the US! Also, more than 28% of people above the age of 18 suffer from high blood pressure and some of them do not even know it yet.

There are several ways through which high blood pressure can be controlled, including the following:

- Keep a healthy diet plan going. This should incorporate a good reduction in sodium intake and fats to keep your arteries safe.

- Be physically active throughout your daily routine.

- Keep a healthy weight without risking your body.

- Keep your consumption of alcoholic beverages in moderation if you have to.

- Take your blood pressure medication if you doctor asks you to use it.

According to *the Seventh Report of the Joint National Committee on Prevention, Detection, Evaluation and Treatment of High Blood Pressure*, the following are the recommended blood pressure levels for adults.

Group	Systolic (mmHg)	Diastolic (mmHg)	Conclusion
Normal	Under 120	Under 80	This is a good rate.
Prehypertension	120 – 139	80 – 89	You are highly likely to develop blood pressure problems. Watch your diet, especially the food you eat and the drinks you consume. Try to be active and lose weight if possible. Consult your doctor in the event that you have diabetes as this may make it worse.
Hypertension	More than 139	More than 89	You are suffering from high blood pressure at this point. Get in touch with your doctor or nurse for help as soon as possible.

The DASH Diet

Did you know that high blood pressure can be very dangerous to your health even if it's just about the normal level? Your normal blood pressure level is supposed to be **120/80 mmHg**. The higher this gets, the greater the risk imposed on your body.

According to the results of research and findings carried out by scientists from the National Heart, Lung, and Blood Institute (NHLBI), your blood pressure can be reduced if you are in a meal plan that is low in saturated fats, cholesterol and total fat content. Apart from that, there should be an emphasis on fruits, vegetables and low-fat milk or dairy products. This is how the DASH Diet came about.

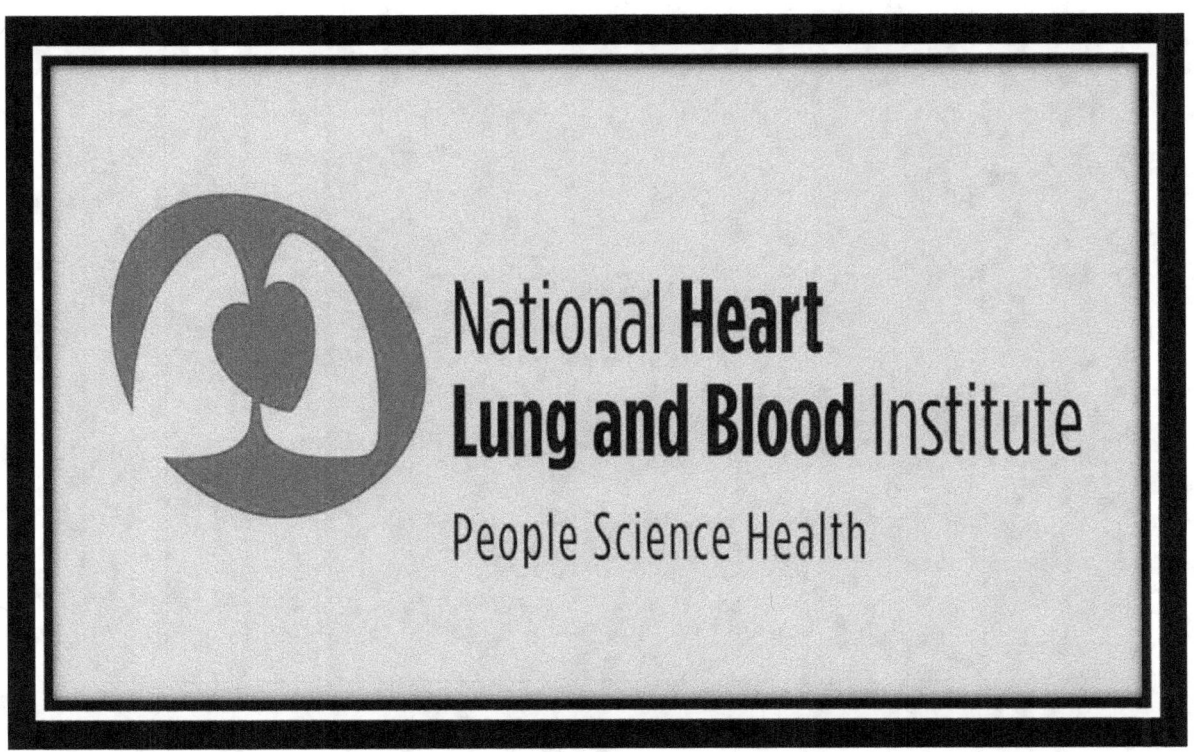

When compared to the average American diet, the DASH diet has plenty of lean bits of content while avoiding massive amounts of red meat, sweets, sugary beverages and anything else with added sugar. It is especially filled with calcium, magnesium and potassium, fiber and protein.

There are many nutritional standards that should be used according to this chart:

Note: This chart is based on the daily DASH diet nutritional targets for a 2100 calorie diet plan.

Total Fat	27% of calories
Saturated Fat	6% of calories
Protein	18% of calories
Carbohydrate	55% of calories
Cholesterol	150 mg
Sodium	2300 mg
Potassium	4700 mg
Calcium	1250 mg
Magnesium	500 mg
Fiber	30 g

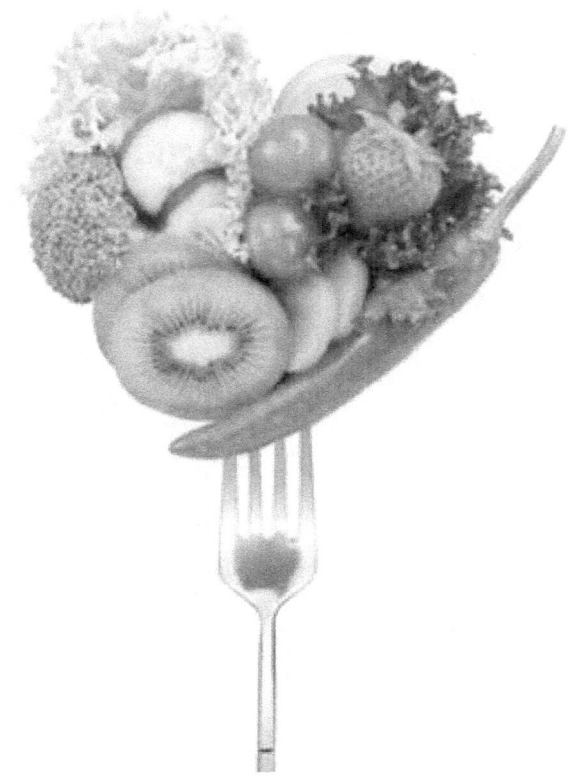

The DASH diet uses healthy guidelines for the heart in an attempt to lower daily saturated fat and cholesterol intake that you might have each day. With this in mind, the emphasis is on increasing the intake of foods that are rich in nutrients to reduce your blood pressure. This is why minerals like potassium and magnesium are included. Besides this, the diet also sets to meet the nutritional requirements specified by the Institute of Medicine.

Initial studies in the DASH Diet

One of the very first DASH diet plans was tested on more than 400 persons whose systolic blood pressure was under 159 mmHg and had a diastolic rate in the range of 80-90 mmHg. More than 25% of the participants had high blood pressure. There were three different diet plans that were used:

- The DASH diet
- A diet plan similar to the normal American diet
- A diet similar to the normal American diet with an inclusion of more fruits and vegetables

Each and every one of the diet plans had 3000 mg of sodium and not a single one of them used any special foods or vegetarian diets.

Based on the studies, the people who partook in the DASH diet and the one with more vegetables and fruits experienced significant reductions in their blood pressure rates.

It is important to also mention that for those who took part in the DASH diet, the blood pressure reduction was rather fast; average results were obtained in 2 weeks.

As it can be noticed, the DASH diet is critical for lowering blood pressure. Apart from that, it was conclusive that irrespective of whichever diet you are on, it is important for you to lower your sodium intake. However, in the event that you are looking for the best results, you should stick to the DASH diet while at the same time working hard to lower your intake of salt and sodium.

Preparing a DASH Meal

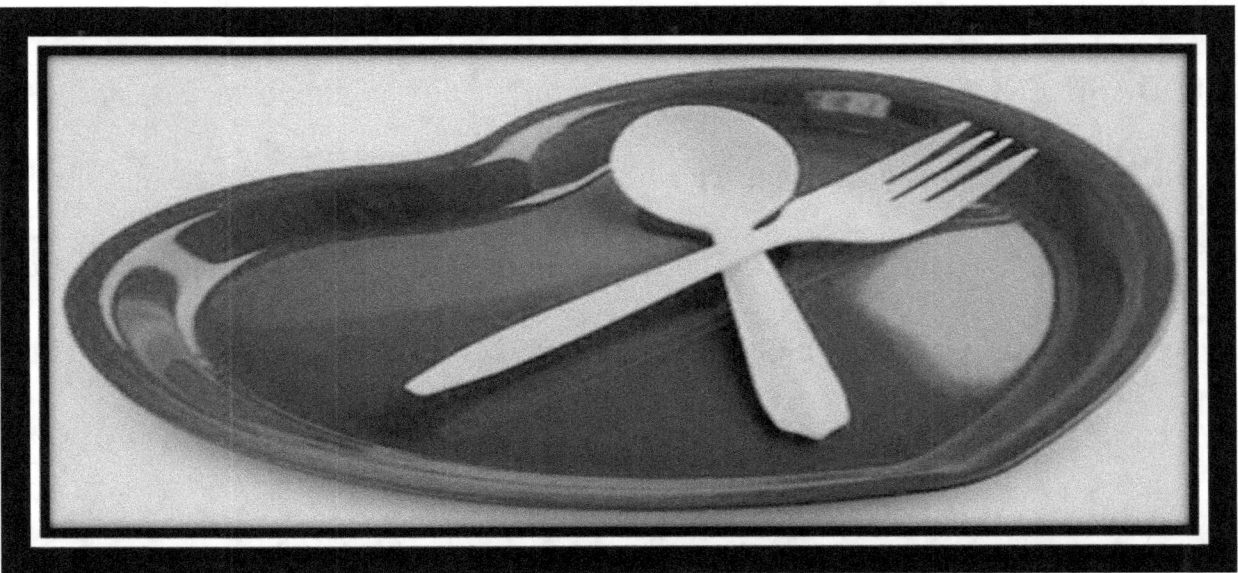

When starting the DASH diet, you have to be aware of the calories that you need to take from time to time. It is important to remember that calorie intake varies from one individual to another and also depends on the daily activities that you'll engage in each day.

There are a number of food groups to take note of when using the DASH diet, especially in terms of the daily recommended servings. When you change your eating habits completely, you will be able to take control of your blood pressure levels. In the event that you are overweight or you are struggling with your weight, you will also keep it in check when you follow the diet plan.

As is the case with most other diet plans, it is recommended that you stop taking alcohol or to at least keep your consumption at moderate levels.

Some exercise is also required to keep you active and to help burning off some of the fat around your body.

The DASH diet is not really defined in terms of any common means, and as a result it is rather broad on what can be done. One of the main reasons for the popularity of the diet lies in the ability to allow those who are suffering from hypertension to lower their blood pressure levels over time, and most importantly to see them get well again. In light of this, you can expect to experience results in a few weeks but the best results will come if you stick with a plan for months on end.

The DASH Diet Eating Plan

In the event that you would like to try out the DASH diet, there are some foods in an eating plan that you should know about. These are available in recommended portions that are healthy for your diet and lifestyle. You should use these considerations when preparing your diet:

Food Category	Recommendation	1/2 Cup Portion Equivalent
Fruits	2 – 2 ½ cups daily	A medium fresh fruit 16 grapes
Vegetables	2 – 2 ½ cups daily	1 cup of low sodium leafy green vegetables
Low fat or fat free dairy	2 – 3 cups daily	8 oz. milk 8 oz. yogurt
Whole grains	6 – 8 ounces daily	1 oz. sliced bread Half a cup of cooked pasta or rice
Lean meat, poultry or fish	6 or less ounces daily	1 egg A pound of cooked beef, chicken or fish
Nuts, seeds & legumes	4 – 5 times a week	Half a cup of cooked dry peas, lentils or beans

Oils	2 – 3 teaspoons daily	A teaspoon of soft margarine A tablespoon of low fat mayonnaise
Added sugar	5 tablespoons a week	A tablespoon of sugar A tablespoon of jelly A cup of lemonade
Sodium	2300 mg per day	1 teaspoon of salt
Alcohol	Sparingly	12 ounces beer 5 ounces wine 1.5 ounce spirits

How to achieve success with the DASH Diet

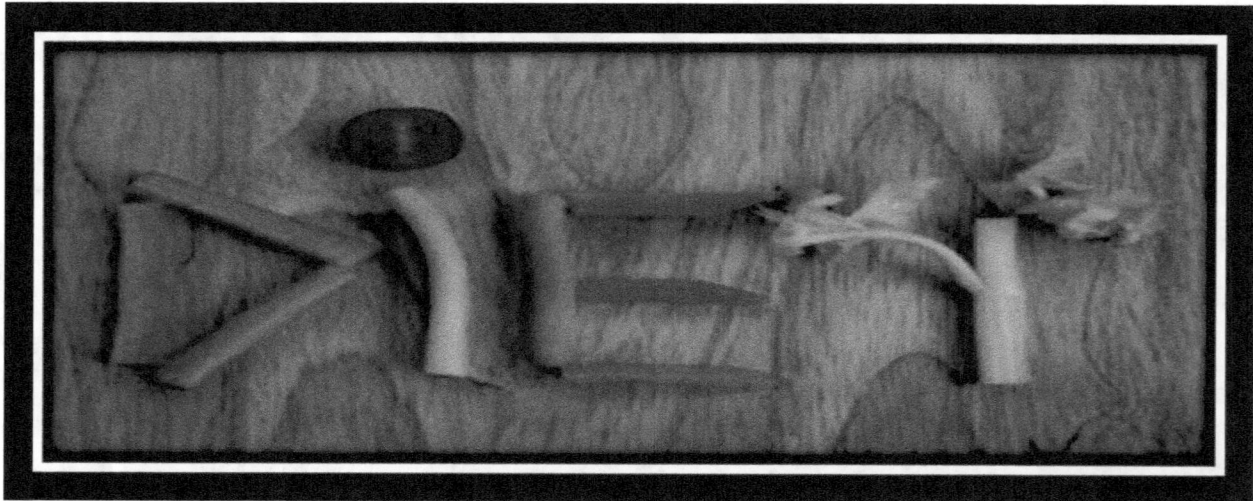

You have to take some time in order for you to get the best results from the diet. For some people, it takes a few days or even two weeks before they start reaping the benefits of the diet. Remember that each and every person has different needs and all of these play different for how the diet works. Your diet and your daily routines can make a real difference.

To achieve success with the DASH diet, you will have to plan out your diet appropriately and accordingly. Always take things one step at a time as there is no need for hurrying. In the event that you are already on a particular diet or you are not practicing any diet at the moment, you will need to be very keen on how you make the switch to the DASH diet.

There is no need for hurrying. As a matter of fact, it is recommended that you switch to the DASH diet gradually so your body can also adapt to the changes and take to the new diet as well as possible. It is important that you start slowly to ease off the pressure. You can even start with a few DASH meals each and every week as you build up the trend.

It will be a lot easier to succeed with the diet in the event that you are already on another diet that includes some of the components of the DASH diet. You'll find it easier to switch in the event that you are already using some of these components.

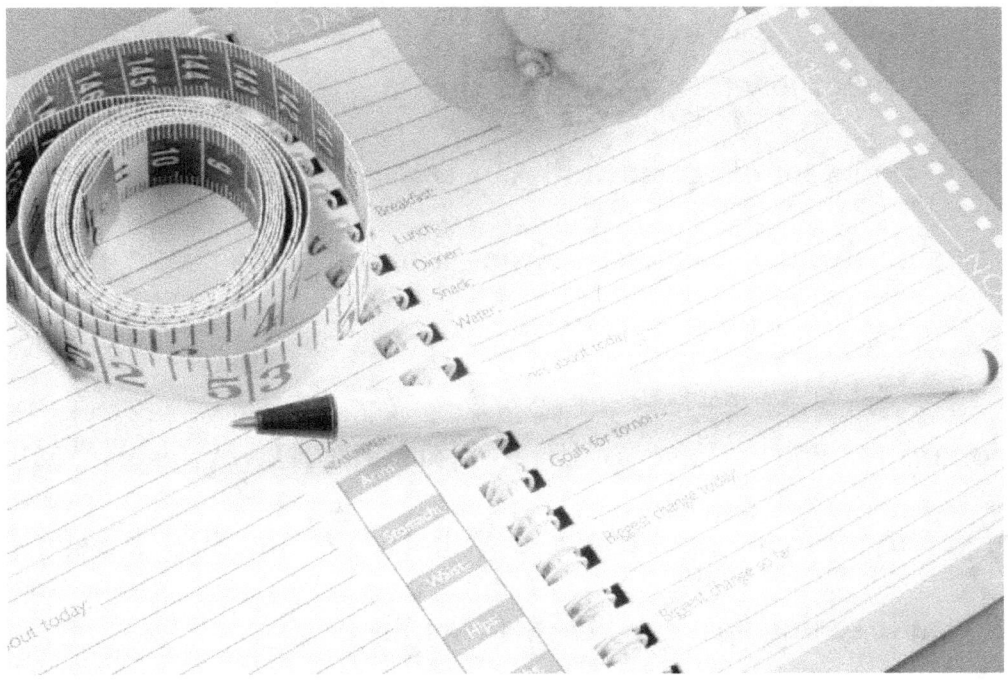

One of the other things that you need to look into is your favorite list of snacks, recipes or even the foods that you eat from time to time. Once you have these in mind, you should set out to include them in the diet plan that you are coming up with. This is very important because it will give you an easier transition from one meal plan to the DASH diet.

It is important for you to take note of which changes to your diet are successes and where you have failed so you'll have something to work with. Take note for the ones that have been successful and feel free to repeat them from time to time because it is these that can make your work easier in terms of adapting to the new diet altogether.

Take note that the DASH diet is something you should be utilizing no matter where you are whether you're in the house or out and about. It does not matter if you are going out of town on a trip or if you are just going out for a quick snack. You can still find a lot of options for your DASH diet no matter how away from home you might be. This therefore means that you also need to look into other alternatives that you can open up to.

It is important for you to have a plan for your diet. Having a plan will make it easier for you to make the right choices. With that in mind, here are some tips that will guide you in setting up a good DASH Diet Plan:

What, when, where and whom do you eat with?

What you eat is very important in this case because knowing in advance what you prefer will make your work easier when looking for options in your diet. This also gives you the perfect understanding of the foods that you can and cannot eat.

Irrespective of what foods you eat or not, take precautions not to fall into any temptations with some really good looking foods that might set you off course.

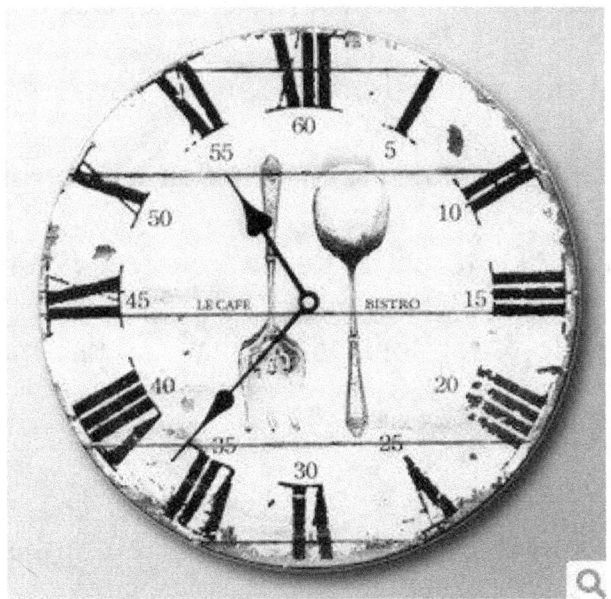

When you eat is also very important. When you are starting out or planning diet it is important that you ensure you understand the times you eat and when you are busy with other things. The importance of this is that it helps you keep tabs on the calories that you eat on a daily basis.

You are not supposed to over-indulge in food. Take note of the number of servings each kind of food you eat that you are supposed to have and try to stick to that. Alternatively, if you already know the number of times that you eat on a daily basis, you can also consider breaking down your meal plan to accommodate your meal times and also make sure that you are able to handle all the pressure that will come with settling on the diet.

Where you eat is as important as what you eat and how much you eat. The place where you have your meals has an influence on the kind of food that you eat from time to time. In the event that you eat your food in a place that is frequented by fast food junkies, you will find yourself bowing to the pressure to try some junk food and so forth. You should get yourself a place to eat where you will have a free will to eat what you would like to eat to make you feel healthy. It might even be recommended that you look for somewhere that has like-minded people on diets whether it's the DASH diet or not.

It's true that there are more restaurants than ever before that are offering healthy dining options. It's a good idea to look around for these places if you have to go someone outside your home to eat. This requires plenty of research on your own but it will be necessary so you'll have a better idea of the right places to visit.

The person with which you eat your food will always have an effect or an influence on so many elements of the food that you eat. If you are surrounded by people who eat a lot then you might end up eating a lot too. This might start off as a dare only to turn into a habit. Therefore, you need to ensure that you eat with people who have positive energies about them wherever they go. Make sure that you eat with people who can support you as you start your new diet and stand by you. Remember that when you are switching to the DASH diet and ditching your old diet, you will be making an important life decision that you should not take for granted.

Incorporate the DASH diet in your daily schedule

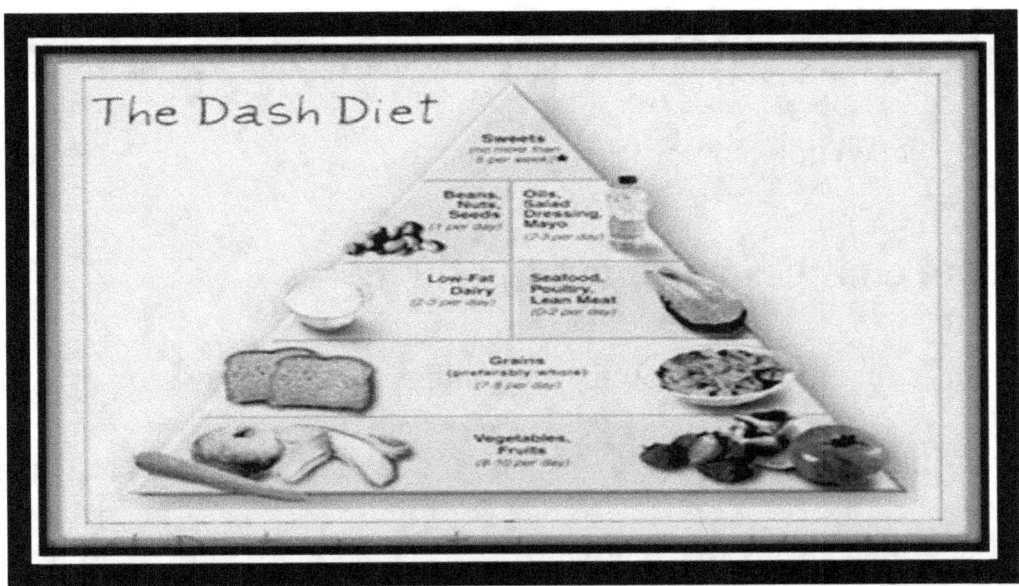

One of the other things that you will need to do is to make the DASH diet part of your daily plan. Your diet is supposed to be part of your life because it makes a significant impact on it.

On the basis of this, you will need to consider incorporating your diet into the routines that you go about, your work and family, even the few times that you set apart to play with friends and family. The importance of this is that you will be getting everyone around you involved in your diet. This is the simplest way of getting the attention and support that you deserve. Do not think of the DASH diet as a diet or meal plan but as a project to set your life in order and to maintain a healthy life. This is where you are supposed to include the foods in the DASH diet that can be considered as snacks and so forth. Remember to try and get anyone around you who will be part of this to understand why they are in it and the importance of the same to you and to them. It is easier to get support from people who understand what you are doing and why you're doing so other than to deal with people who do not know what you are up to.

Anticipate changes and plan for them

Anticipation is one of the most important things that you have to perfect when it comes to trying out a new diet. It is important for you to make sure that you can anticipate and plan ahead for a particular diet that you are on. As is the case with all the other diets out there, you will need to be prepared and ready for the DASH diet and the changes that will come with it.

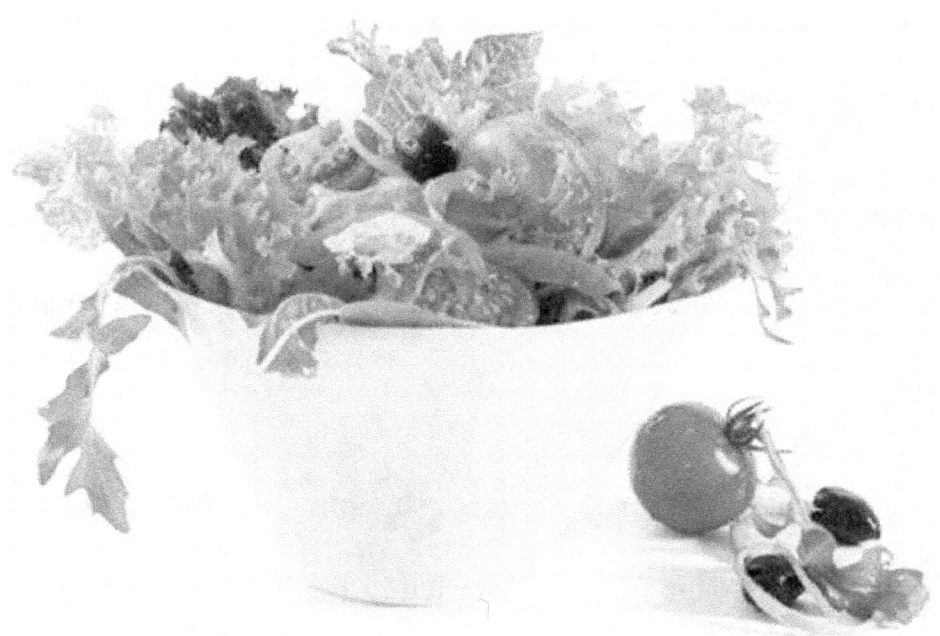

The main reason for doing this is that you will need to be prepared for any changes in the manner you eat or how you eat or even what you eat. It is important to take note of this so that you can look into any allergies other conditions that you will need to take note of before you start or continue with the diet. Remember to speak to your doctor or your nutritionist before you set out on any diet so that you can get the best professional guidance on the right course of action.

Planning Tools

Planning tools are very essential to your success with the diet. There are a number of planning tools that you can use, including the *Weekly Meal Planner* or the *Daily DASH Tracker*, two common and effective tools. You need a planner to ensure that you follow a given path and that you can stick to it. When you do this it will be easier for you to determine the best foods available for you and when to take them. It will also create a sense of.

It is also important that you follow the meal plans accordingly. For instance, you can't just have snacks as they can keep you off-track. Follow your plan strictly for the best results.

You need to know how to make a good shopping list too. Your shopping list should be your guide to shopping appropriately for the food that you will use on your diet. As long as you know what you need to buy, you will not need to worry about buying food that you will not need to eat.

Shopping for DASH Diet foods

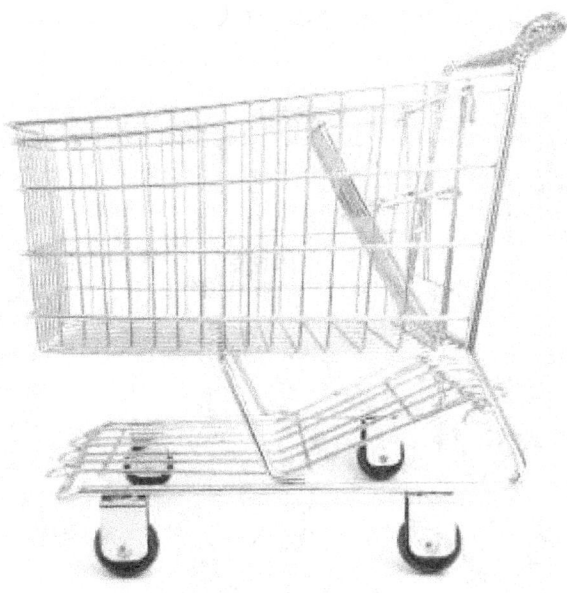

You will come to realize that shopping is easy when you have a shopping list and you know what you're supposed to get. This couldn't be truer for grocery shopping. It's easy and cheap to buy foods when you already have a plan.

You look into the meals that you are planning to have in the course of the week before shopping. This is so you can go out and buy these in advance. You should ensure that you have the ingredients that you need in your shopping list before you set out. This will also make it easier for you to avoid impulse purchases.

The following are some of the important tips that you are supposed to have in mind when you are drawing up your shopping list:

Think in terms of seasonal vegetables and fruits.

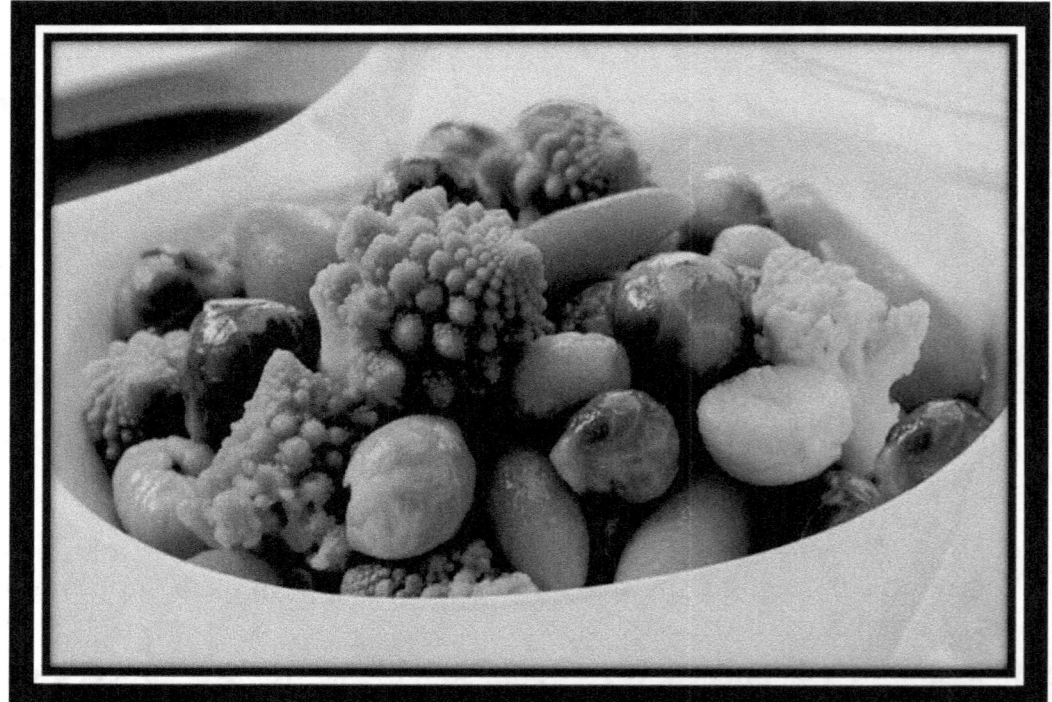

It is important that you get your meals in check in as far as the fruits and vegetables are concerned. You should especially be aware of when different fruits and vegetables might be available so you can prepare your diet during the right times. This is important because there are some fruits and vegetables that are not usually available in stores when they are out of season, and as such you would not want to backtrack on your diet because your fruits or vegetables are not available in the groceries.

Whole grain foods have to be factored into the mix as well.

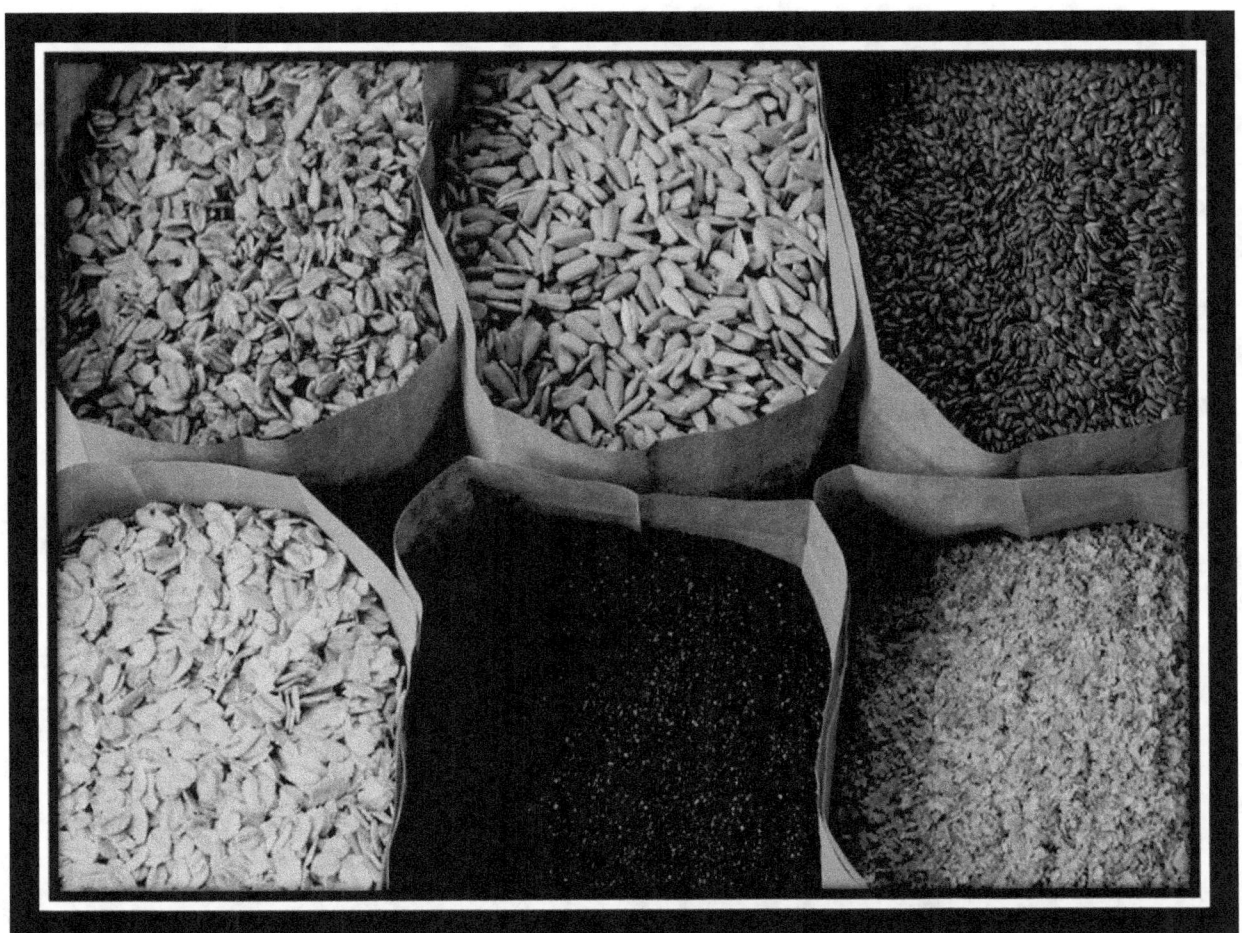

You should draw up a good shopping list that has plenty of whole grain foods.

Some of the foods to consider when drafting your list include whole wheat pasta, whole wheat bread (make sure it is 100% whole wheat), barley, brown rice and quinoa.

These make for a good addition to your shopping list as you'll target the grains portion of your diet.

Protein and fiber content are two critical points to use in your diet.

Your diet needs beans, peas, lentils and many other fiber-rich foods. In fact, these foods can contain protein just as well.

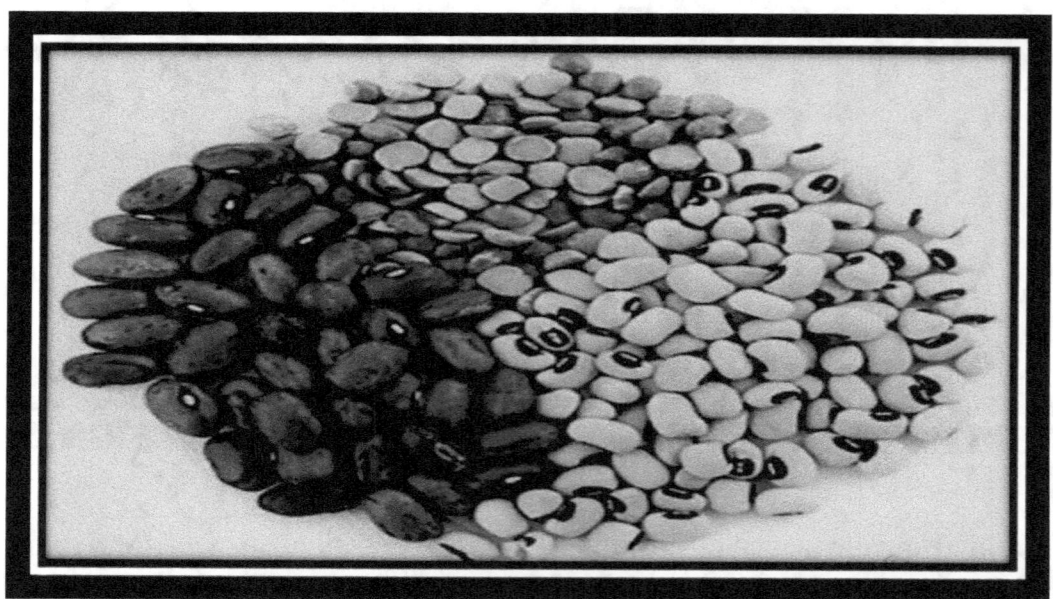

Other foods that you need to add to your shopping list include the following:

- Lean meats, tofu, seafood and poultry that has its skin removed

- Fat-free dairy products or low fat products if fat-free isn't available

- Canned vegetables (low in sodium), tomato sauce, soup and broth, or beans

- Low calorie beverages

- Herbal tea

- Mineral water

- Vegetable juice

- Pure natural fruit juice, made from 100% fruit juice with no additive chemicals

- Condiments and dressings with low sodium content

The following shopping list should guide you on some of the foods that you can consider the next time you are making plans for your own:

Vegetables	Fruit	Dairy	Condiments	Frozen Food
Artichokes	Apples	Yogurt	Vinegar	Waffles
Asparagus	Mangoes	Kefir	Sun-dried	Veggie
Beets	Pineapples	Sour cream	tomatoes	burgers
Bell Pepper	Raisins	Margarine	Salad dressing	Pancakes
Broccoli	Prunes	Cheese	Pesto	Vegetables
Brussels	Apricots	Buttermilk	Canola oil	Fruit juice
Sprout	Bananas	Mozzarella	Sesame	Fruits
Mushrooms	Cherries		Mayonnaise	Chicken breast
Eggplant	Grapes		Hummus	Fish fillets
Corn	Kiwi fruit		Chili sauce	French toast
Cucumber	Papaya			
Carrots	Plums			
Cabbage				

Packaged Snacks	Meat, Seafood, Poultry, Soy	Canned Food	Nuts & Seeds	Bread
Pretzels	Tofu	Tomato paste	Walnuts	Tortilla
Dried fruit	Tempeh	Tomato sauce	Soy nuts	Pizza crust
Crackers	Salmon	Tomatoes	Seeds	Pita
Popcorn	Shrimp	Soup	Almonds	Bagel
	Eggs	Salmon	Cashews	English
	Beef (lean)	Tuna	Hazelnuts	muffins
	Pork	Chilies	Pecans	Bread
	(tenderloin)	Broth	Seeds	
	Chicken	Beans	Peanuts	
	Turkey	Lentils	Nut butter	
		Applesauce		

Cereal	Grains	Beverages	Herbs & Spices
Oats	Wild rice	Fruit juice (100%)	Dill
Muesli	Kamut	Vegetable juice	Ginger
Bran cereal	Spelt	Sparkling water	Basil
Low fat granola	Pasta	Herbal tea	Chilli flakes
Whole grain cereal	Quinoa		Cilantro
	Oats		Cumin
	Barley		Garlic
	Brown rice		Mint
	Bulgur		Oregano
	Kasha		Paprika
			Nutmeg
			Curry powder
			Cloves
			Cinnamon

A guide to DASH Meals

Switching to the DASH diet can be a very simple thing yet for some people it can be quite the challenge. In the face of this, it will be easier for you to make the required steps towards your DASH diet as long as you have a guideline on the best foods that should make up your meals.

It is highly likely that you are already eating some of the components of the DASH diet, including things like fruits and vegetables. You have to make changes when you enter the DASH diet though. For instance, you are supposed to increase your overall intake of certain kinds of food like the fruits and vegetables.

The best way to start is to focus on one meal at a time and then build off of it.

The following are some of the solutions that you can consider for your meals.

Breakfast Options

You can prepare a cappuccino or a latte as long as you use low fat milk. This may include either 1 or 2% milk or skim milk, a form of milk that contains little to no fat. Use as little fat as possible in order to get the best results out of your diet.

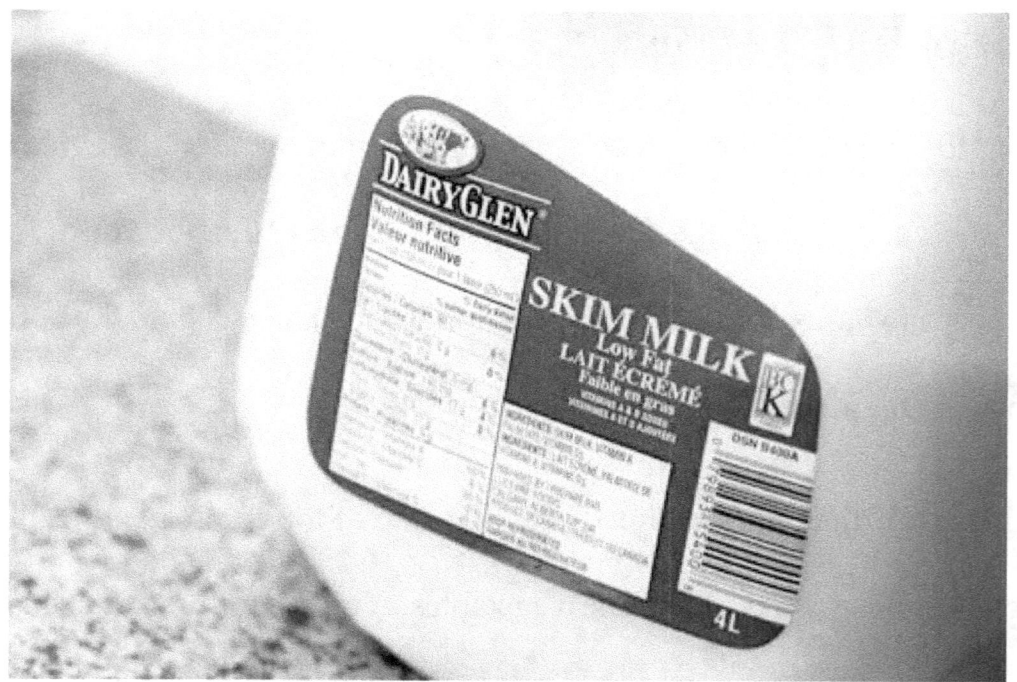

Prepare an easy smoothie with 100% natural fruit juice, yogurt (low fat) and any frozen fruit (preferably a banana).

If you are making an omelet, you can add some chopped vegetables to it. This will also work with scrambled eggs.

Prepare an English muffin and top it up with tomato sauce. You can also use a slice of cheese (low fat) to add to this.

Use nut butter if you are eating whole grain toast. Alternatively, you can also top it up with some raisins, pears or bananas.

For those who love to have oatmeal in the morning, you can make it with low fat milk instead of water. You can also add in some nuts or sliced fruits as toppings.

Lunch Options

The following are some of the best and easiest-to-prepare options that you have for lunch:

If you are having a sandwich for lunch, you can add in low fat cheese. This will give you a boost of calcium and protein.

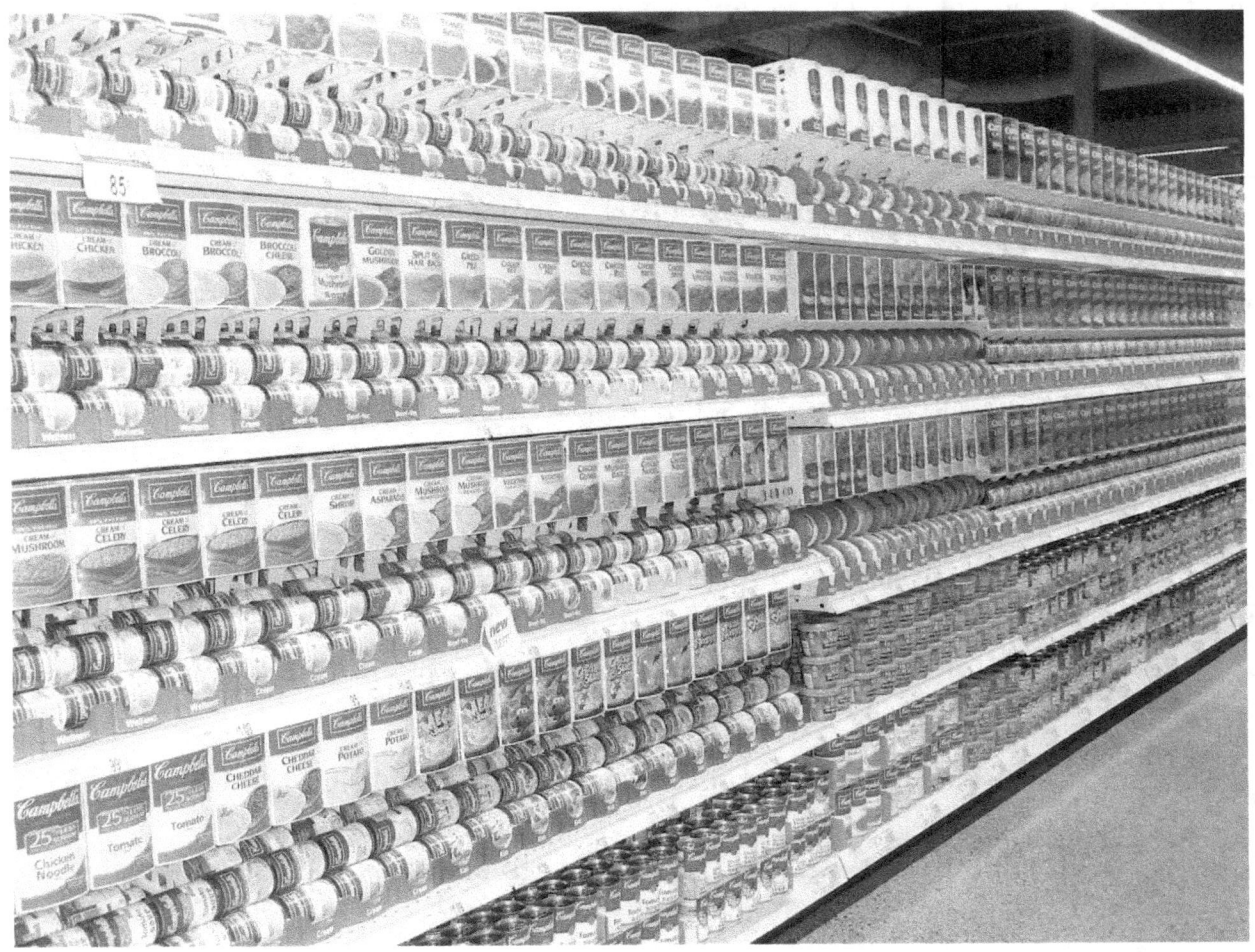

For those who make soups or buy canned soups, you can try adding in frozen vegetables or fresh ones. Of course, it's a good idea to try and find low-sodium variants of many of these soups. You can find out which ones have low amounts of sodium in them by looking at the labels. For instance, the soups in the picture above that feature green labels are the ones that have less sodium in them.

You can make soup with low fat milk instead of cream or water. Cream contains too much fat and should be controlled.

You can always use like mandarin orange slices, dried fruit, pineapples and grapes to top up your salads. Diced apples, seeds and crunchy nuts are also good alternatives.

Try to avoid soft drinks. You can consider using low fat milk or fat free milk instead.

It is better to prepare your own sandwiches instead of buying them. When you prepare your own sandwiches, you need to make sure that you use whole grain bread as it is rich in fiber. In addition, you won't have to worry about the processed stuff that comes with some ready-made sandwiches that you could buy.

When preparing sandwiches, you need to pack them with a lot of vegetables. You can consider adding in things like grated carrots, tomatoes, mixed greens and peppers.

During lunch, always make sure that you are at the salad section and try some of the healthy stuff there like bean soup, lentils or any vegetable broth available.

Dinner Options

For dinner, it is recommended that you try some of the following options in the event that you want to make sure that you are on a good DASH Diet:

Have some steamed vegetables that aren't fried.

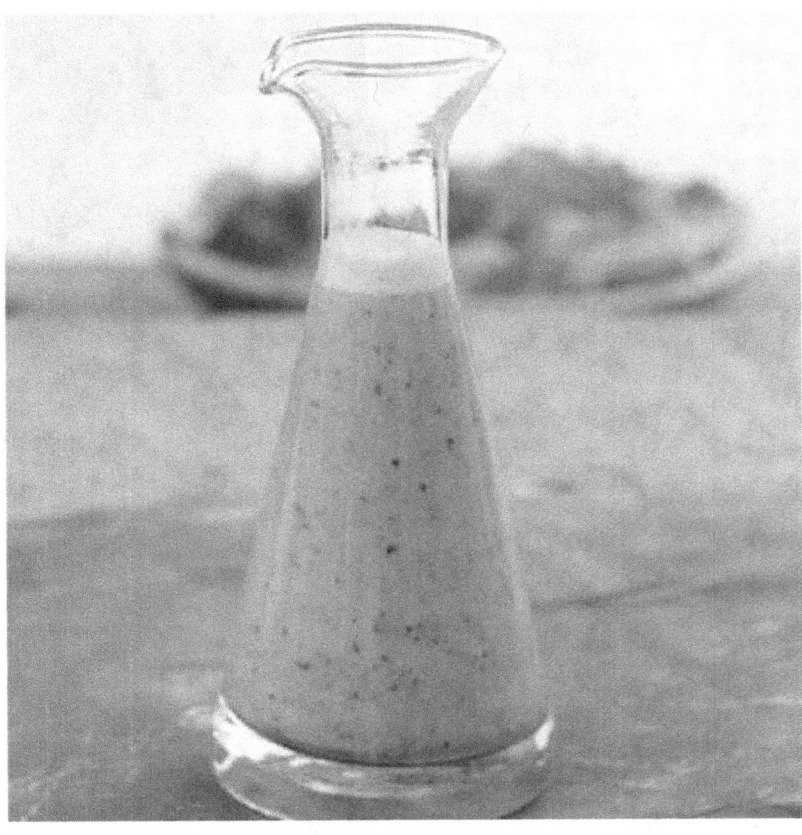

You can season with vinaigrette dressing for flavoring.

Always begin your meals with green salads. Leafy green vegetables with fiber should help you to keep yourself healthy and safe.

Consider progressively removing meat from your recipes for a vegetarian diet. It's best to do this gradually so you don't feel upset or irritated while on your diet.

Dessert Options

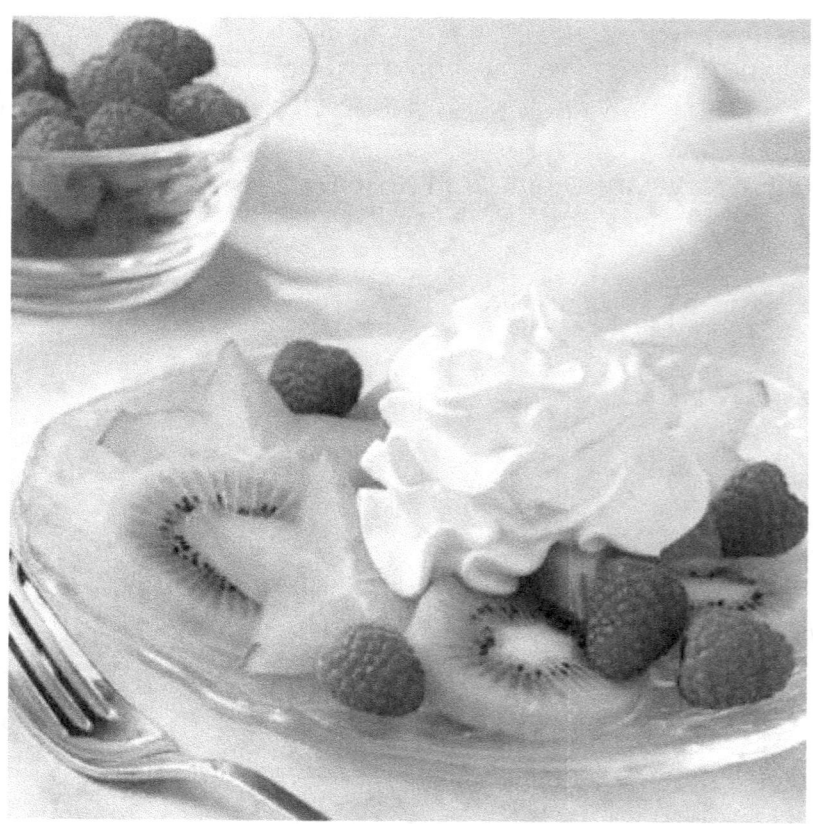

Whatever you do, always try to make sure your dessert has loads of fruits. This is a sure way to stay healthy without much of an effort.

You can also consider baked apples, bananas or even pears and mix them with low fat yogurt.

When berries are in season, you can take advantage of this and top them with vanilla yogurt. You can also sprinkle sliced almonds on them for more flavors.

Frequently Asked Questions

When it comes to the DASH Diet, there are a number of questions that people usually need to answer over time. This is a common feature in all diets because people usually need to make sure that whatever diets they are starting on will be worth their time and investment.

The other reason why people raise a lot of questions is because they need to make sure they are making the right decision when looking for a diet plan. The following are some of the most common questions that are addressed towards the DASH Diet. There are many good answers with regards to how the whole process should work.

How does it work?

The DASH diet works in a very simple. The main pretext is to make you cut down on the amount of salt that you eat from time to time. However, apart from that you will need to select the calories that you need to eat on a daily basis and ensure that your diet focuses on a lot of fruits and vegetables.

Can you lose weight with the DASH Diet?

Take note that the DASH diet is not a diet that is designed to help in losing weight, but the main aim is to prevent hypertension or help remedy a blood pressure condition that you might already be developing without your knowledge.

This does not mean that you cannot cut down some pounds in the process. It is highly likely that you will be able to lose some weight, especially when you work on a good diet plan with a calorie deficit.

Are there any benefits to the heart?

Yes! There are many studies that have been carried out into the diet to confirm some of the benefits. The DASH diet can help you lower your blood pressure. Remember that when your blood pressure is so high, you will run the risk of heart problems, potential heart failure or even a stroke.

The diet has also been documented to lower bad cholesterol (LDL) and increase good cholesterol (HDL) in the body. This also goes a long way in preventing heart disease.

Generally, this is one of the best diets that has ever been recommended by the medical society especially with the focus on the safety of the heart.

What about diabetes?

There are a number of studies that have been carried out which have shown good results with regards to diabetes. For this reason therefore there are dieticians who recommend the diet for those who are worried about diabetes. It is also important to note that the American Diabetes Association has also gone on to give a recommendation to the DASH Diet, making it a commendable option for you.

Should I worry about any health risks?

There are no known risks related to the DASH Diet in terms of what can happen. However, it is always reasonable for you to consult your doctor or nutritionist before you set out on any new diet plan.

Does the diet meet the recommended government diet guidelines?

Indeed, the DASH diet does meet the required guidelines set by the government and other authorities. This can be outlined as below:

Fat: The government recommends 20 – 35% of calories of total fat on a daily basis with a limit of 10% for saturated fat.

The diet also is within the recommended limits for protein, carbohydrates and salt.

Some of the other benefits that you have to take note of include the use of fiber, potassium, calcium, Vitamin B – 12 and Vitamin D.

Also, take note that you do not need any supplement with this diet whatsoever.

Is it easy to follow?

It is very easy for anyone who is interested to follow the DASH diet. This is because it does not restrict you by making you quit any foods that you often eat. As a matter of fact, you will even be able to consume alcoholic beverages albeit in moderation.

It is understandable that quitting sugary and fatty foods completely can be a nightmare to a lot of people, and this is why integrating the DASH diet into your meal plan is so easy to keep you from struggling with it.

Is it a convenient diet?

There are a lot of options that you can use in terms of making your recipes. You do not have to worry about making the diet. It will be so easy for you to keep this diet as it is very convenient for you.

Is it satisfactory?

When you are eating, nutritionists and other experts usually recommend that you are satisfied with regards to what you want to eat. Through the DASH diet, you will not have to worry about satiety especially because you will be eating so much lean protein, vegetables and fiber fruits. Therefore, you should eat to your satisfaction even when you have reduced your calorie intake.

Taste

One of the things that you will have to adjust to is the feeling of not having to eat your popcorn and other junk foods. However, you need to get accustomed to the taste of herbs and spices as these will make up a huge part of your diet.

What about other dietary preferences?

You do not have to worry if you're already on another diet. The DASH Diet can be used by anyone. All you have to do is to make sure you speak to your doctor before you can set out on this diet. Your doctor can give you more guidance on this.

You can use the diet even if you are on a gluten free, vegetarian, vegan, halal, kosher or low salt diet.

Is exercise necessary?

Exercise and dieting go hand in hand. It is recommended that you exercise often especially when you are looking to get the best out of your diet plan. If you are keen on losing some weight, this will be a very good alternative for you.

I am lactose intolerant; can I use the DASH Diet?

There are a lot of people who cannot tolerate lactose yet they are still able to use yogurt, cheese and heated milk products. What you need to do is to use substitutes that contain a good amount of calcium and vitamin D as the original foods from which they are derived. Some of the substitutes include almond and soy.

If you have an issue with the protein in cow milk, you can also try goat milk. You can also consider other cultured milk products in the event that your body is sensitive to milk protein or lactose.

I have celiac disease and want to follow the DASH Diet. What can I do?

Those with celiac disease usually avoid foods with gluten. However, this does not mean that you cannot use the DASH Diet. All you will need to do is to substitute any of the grains with foods that are approved for a gluten-free diet and you will be able to use the DASH Diet.

Is the diet low in fat?

The DASH diet is indeed low in fats; the fats that you take in are fats that are healthy to the heart.

Is the diet high on fiber?

The fiber content of the DASH diet is commendable and should really help you out.

Are there vegan or vegetarian versions of the DASH diet?

In the event that you are a vegetarian or you are practicing a vegan diet, there are a number of foods that will make your eating plan worthwhile. The DASH diet is composed of beans, nuts and seeds and at the same time has substitutions for meat, poultry and even fish.

Take note that the DASH diet is designed to offer you the benefits you get from vegan diets in as far as reducing heart pressure is concerned.

Can I make substitutions in the event that I do not like some of the foods in the DASH diet books?

The diet is a very flexible one and you are free to make substitutions to any of the foods that make up the diet plan. The only thing that you will need to be aware of is to keep track of the nutrient content of the foods that you are substituting. A lot of diet books also come with substitute foods that you can use and their contents as far as minerals are concerned.

Sea salt or regular salt - which one should I use?

It is notable that a lot of sea salts are usually low on sodium as compared to regular salts. However, you have to take note that even sea salt can still contribute to an increase in the sodium content in your diet.

Instead of using salt to season your food, you need to try and learn how to season your food through a number of available options.

I want to use salt substitutes that have potassium chloride. What can I do here?

Before you do this, it is important that you consult your doctor first. The reason for this is because there are a number of medications that will make you retain potassium. This could be dangerous to your body over time. Therefore, you have to make sure that you only use this with your doctor's consent.

DASH Diet Recipes

Here are some really amazing DASH diet recipes that will guide you on how to prepare some really healthy meals and also keep your health in check. These are recipes that you can use on a daily or weekly basis to keep your heart healthy.

Note: The recipes are for a 1500 mg-per-day sodium intake level.

Skinless Chicken Salad

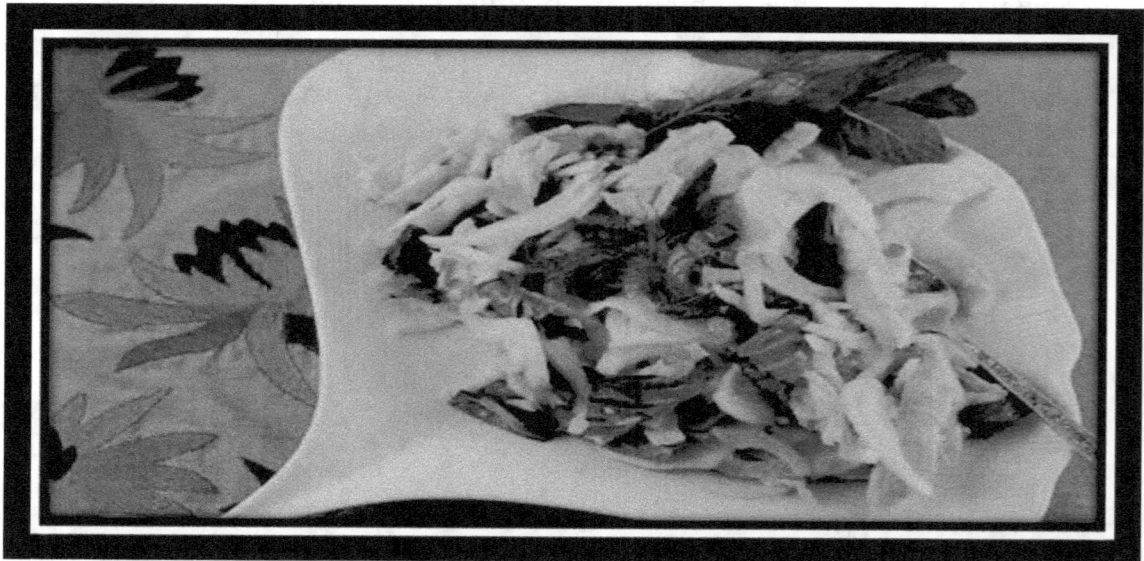

This meal serves 5

Ingredients

3 tablespoons low fat Mayonnaise

1/8 teaspoon salt (it is recommended that you omit this)

3 cups cooked cubed skinless chicken breast

1/2 teaspoon onion powder

1 tablespoon of Lemon Juice

1/4 cup chopped Celery

Preparation Method

Bake the chicken at hand.

Cut the chicken into small cube like pieces.

Refrigerate the chicken cubes.

Combine all the other ingredients together in a different bowl.

Add the refrigerated chicken (chilled) and mix properly.

Serve.

The nutrient content of this meal is as follows:

Total Fat	6 g
Saturated Fat	2 g
Protein	27 g
Calories	176
Carbohydrate	2 g
Cholesterol	77 mg
Sodium	179 mg
Potassium	236 mg
Calcium	16 mg
Magnesium	25 mg
Fiber	0 g

Spaghetti Sauce for Vegetarians

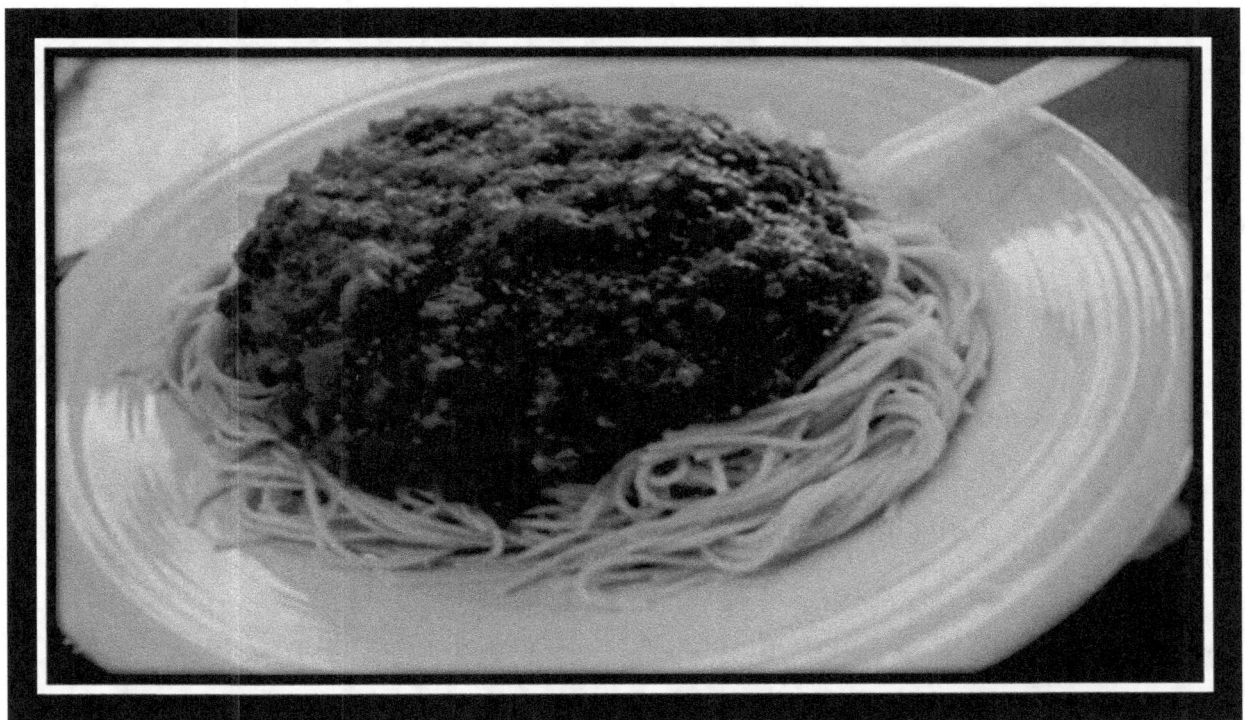

This meal serves 6 and takes 1 hour to complete

Ingredients

1 cup of water

2 chopped medium tomatoes

2 tablespoons olive oil

2 small chopped onions

1 tablespoon dried basil

Low sodium tomato paste (1 can)

Tomato sauce (1 8 oz can)

1 tablespoon dried oregano

1 1/2 cups sliced zucchini

3 chopped garlic cloves

Preparation method

Take a medium skillet and heat oil inside.

Saute the zucchini, garlic and onions for 5 minutes at a medium setting.

Add all the other ingredients and cover then simmer for 40 minutes.

Serve with spaghetti.

The nutrient content of this meal is as follows:

Total Fat	5 g
Saturated Fat	1 g
Protein	3 g
Carbohydrate	15 g
Cholesterol	0 mg
Sodium	479 mg
Calories	105
Potassium	686 mg
Calcium	49 mg
Magnesium	35 mg
Fiber	4 g

Baba Ghanoush

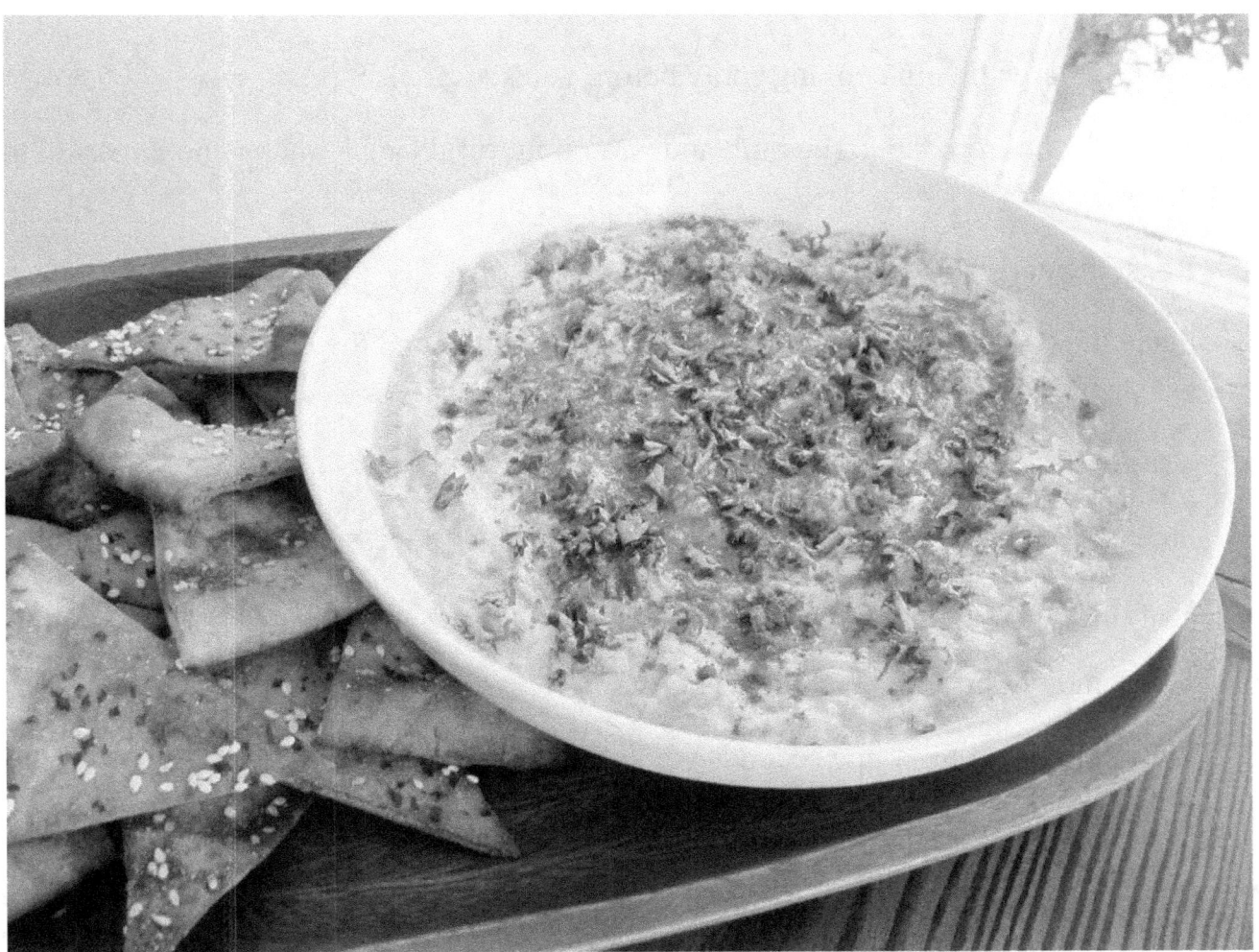

Serves 4 and takes 40 minutes

Ingredients

1 garlic bulb

2 sliced eggplants

1 red bell pepper

4 tablespoons of fresh lemon juice

1 tablespoon of olive oil

1 tablespoon of black pepper

2 flatbread or pita rounds

Preparation Method

Spray your grill with cooking spray before you start to heat it up.

Slice the top from the garlic bulb and wrap it in foil. Place it on the cooler part of the grill.

Roast the garlic bulb for 25 minutes.

Place the eggplant slices, preferably cut horizontally, and the bell pepper to the hot side.

Grill for 2-3 minutes on each side.

Squeeze out your roasted garlic and add it in a food processor.

Mix the finished eggplant and pepper in the processor.

Add lemon juice and olive oil and stir it in.

Warm the bread for a few seconds while flipping it midway through.

The bread can be broken up if desired.

Serve immediately. Lettuce or oregano may be added to the top as a garnish.

The nutrient content of this meal is as follows:

Total Fat	4 g
Saturated Fat	0.6 g
Protein	4 g
Carbohydrate	25 g
Cholesterol	0 mg
Sodium	160 mg
Calories	148
Potassium	4 mg
Calcium	2 mg
Magnesium	1 mg
Fiber	3 g

Vinaigrette Salad Dressing

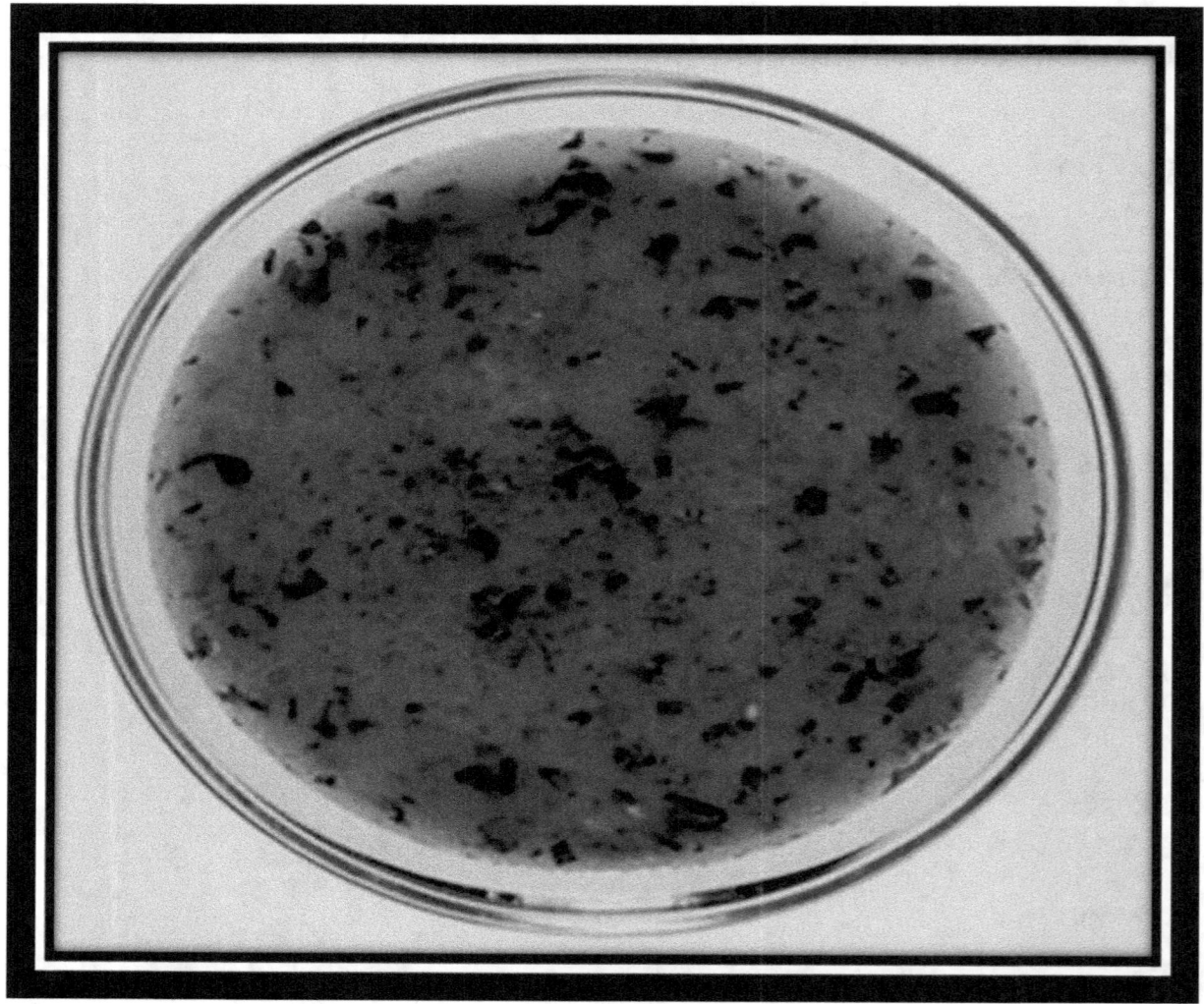

Serves 4 and takes 30 minutes to cook

Ingredients

1/4 teaspoon black pepper

1 garlic bulb

1/2 cup of water

1 tablespoon virgin olive oil

1 tablespoon vinegar (red wine)

1/4 teaspoon honey

Preparation Method

Cover the garlic in a saucepan with water.

Boil the water for 15 minutes then lower the heat and simmer until all the garlic is so tender.

Remove some of the liquid until you have only 2-3 tablespoons and heat for 3-4 minutes.

Transfer the contents to another bowl then mash the garlic.

Whisk in vinegar with some seasoning and some oil.

Serve.

The nutrient content of this meal is as follows:

Total Fat	3 g
Saturated Fat	1 g
Protein	0 g
Carbohydrate	1 g
Cholesterol	0 mg
Sodium	1 mg
Calories	33
Potassium	6 mg
Calcium	3 mg
Magnesium	1 mg
Fiber	0 g

Potato Salad

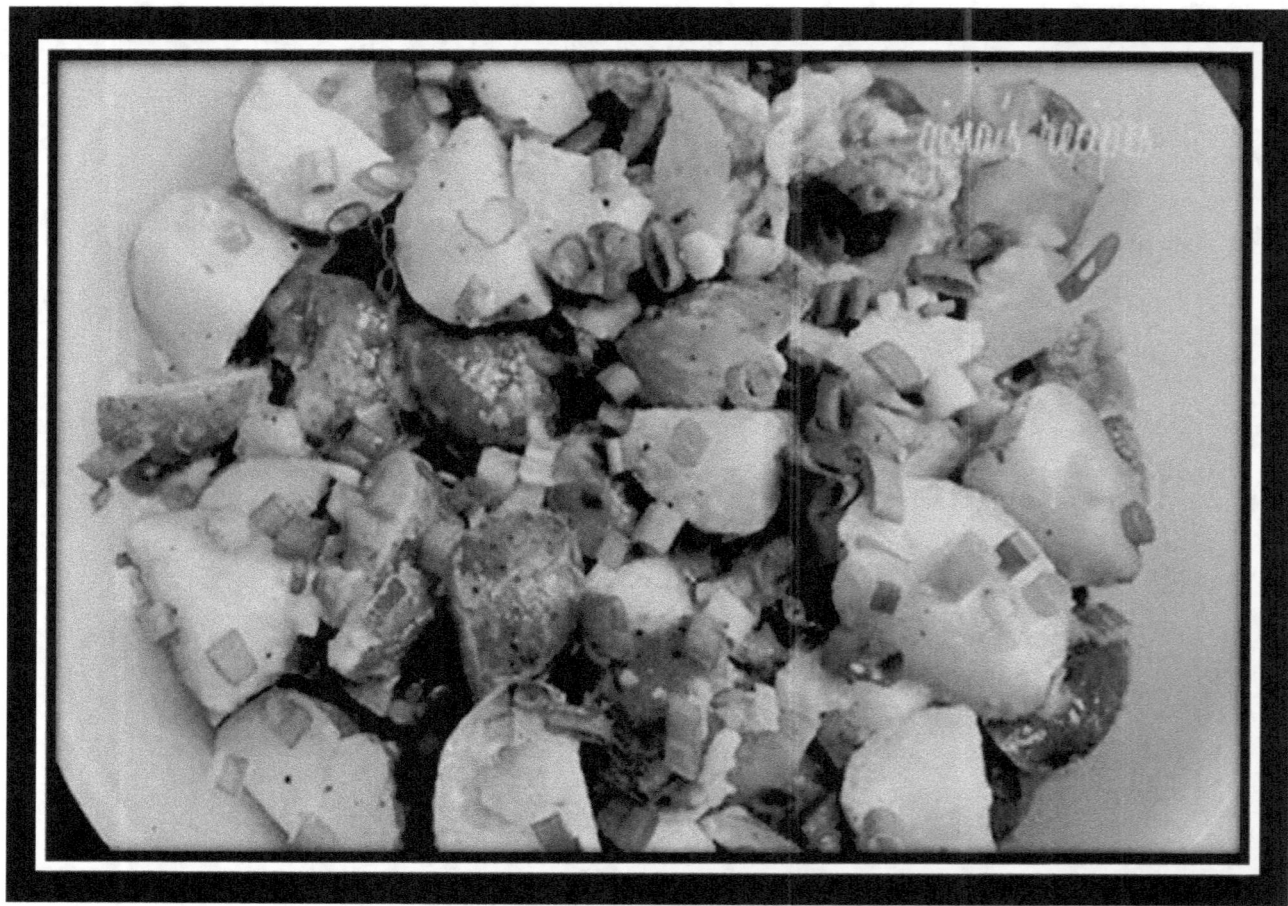

Serves 5 and takes 1 hour

Ingredients

1 teaspoon dried dill weed

5 cups of potatoes (15 small potatoes)

2 tablespoons olive oil

1/4 teaspoon black pepper

1/4 cup chopped green onions

Preparation Method

Clean the potatoes properly and run them through water.

Boil the potatoes until they become soft and tender; this takes roughly 15 - 20 minutes.

Drain and allow the potatoes to cool down.

Cut the potatoes into 4 quarters then mix in the onions, spices and olive oil.

The nutrient content of this meal is as follows:

Total Fat	6 g
Saturated Fat	1 g
Protein	4 g
Carbohydrate	34 g
Cholesterol	0 mg
Sodium	17 mg
Calories	196
Potassium	861 mg
Calcium	31 mg
Magnesium	46 mg
Fiber	4 g

Spanish Rice with Chicken

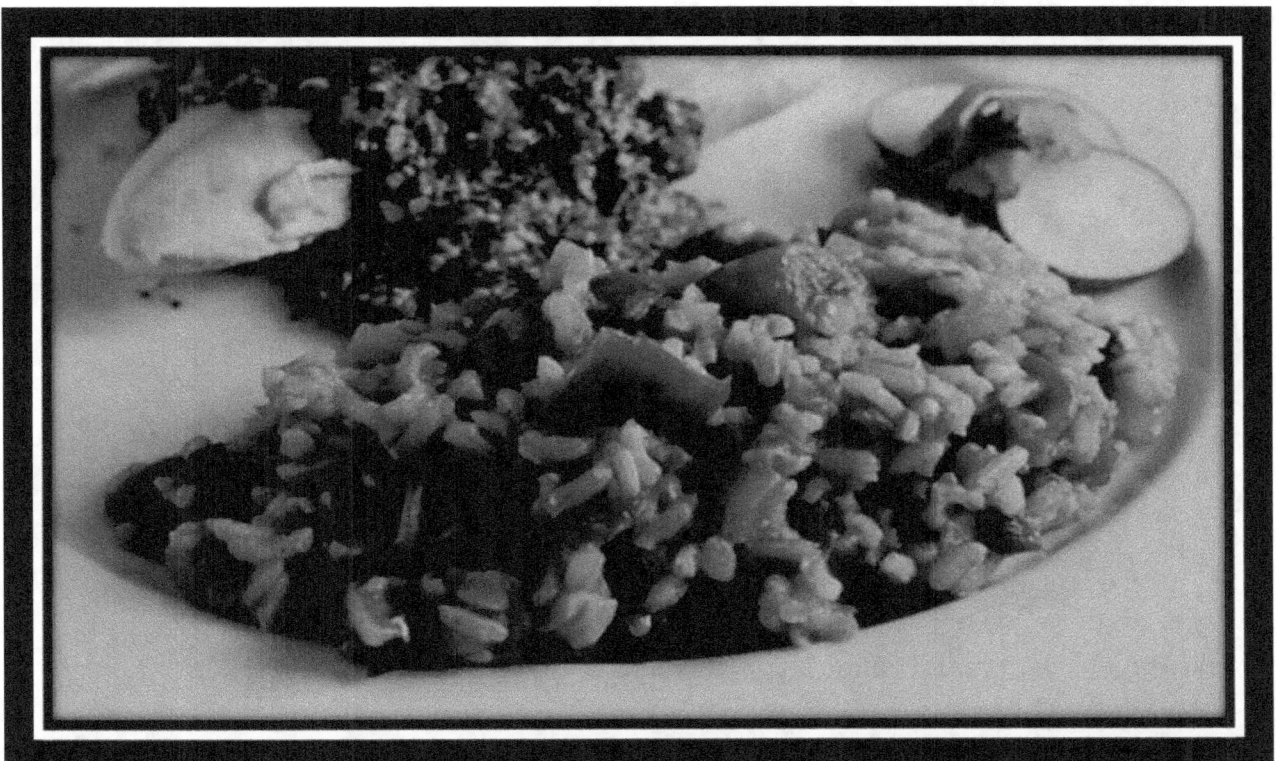

Serves 5 with a time of 20 minutes to prepare

Ingredients

3 cups diced and cooked chicken breasts without the skin and bones

5 cups brown rice cooked in unsalted water

1 teaspoon minced garlic

1/2 teaspoon black pepper

1 cup chopped onions

3/4 cup green pepper

1 teaspoon chopped parsley

2 teaspoons vegetable oil

Tomato sauce (1 can)

Preparation Method

Saute the pepper and onions in a skillet on medium heat for 5 minutes.

Add spices and tomato sauce and then heat properly.

Add the chicken and rice and heat properly.

Serve.

The nutrient content of this meal is as follows:

Total Fat	8 g
Saturated Fat	2 g
Protein	35 g
Carbohydrate	52 g
Cholesterol	80 mg
Sodium	341 mg
Calories	428
Potassium	545 mg
Calcium	50 mg
Magnesium	122 mg
Fiber	8 g

Grilled Pineapple

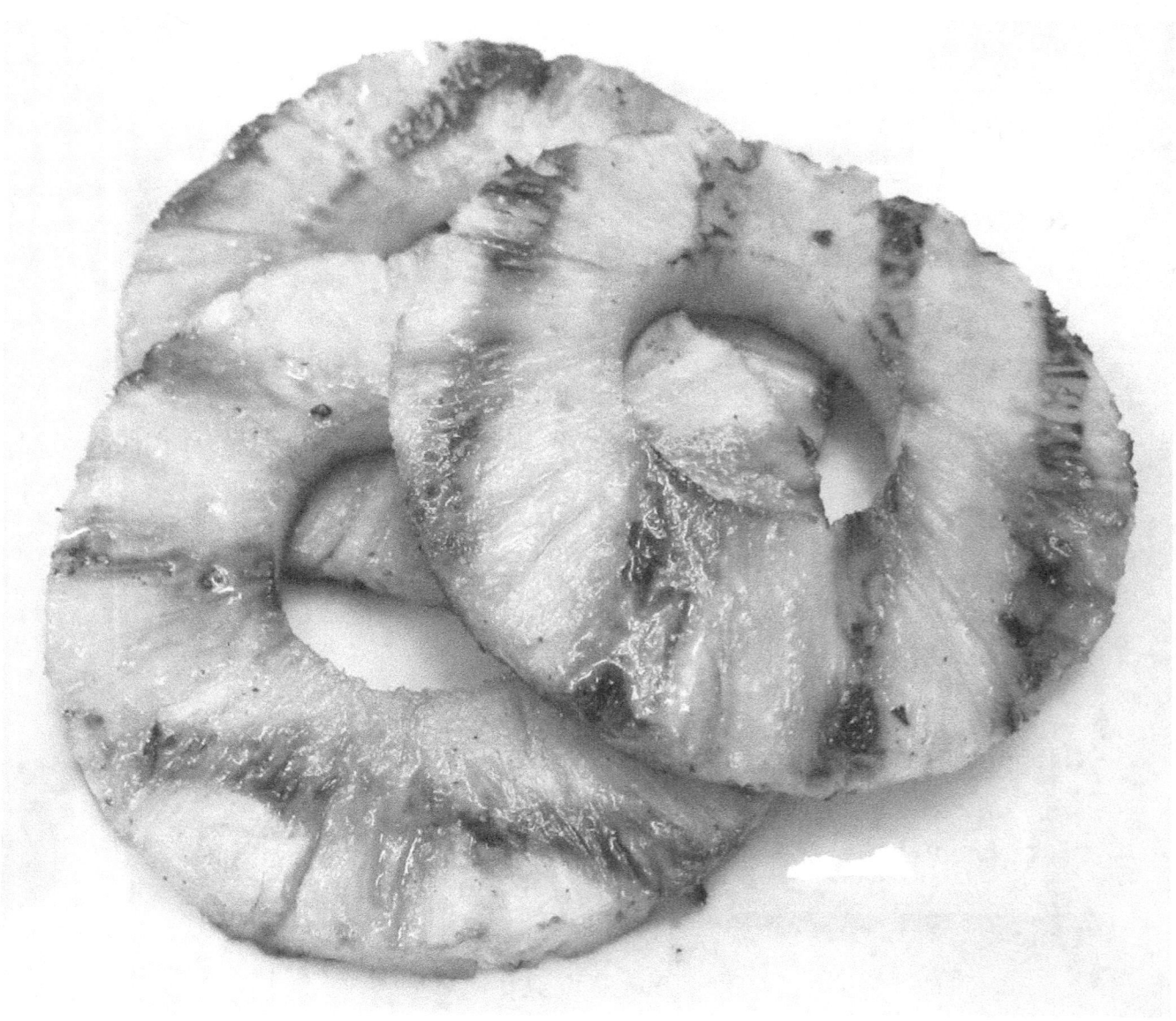

Serves 8, requires 15 minutes

Ingredients

1 firm pineapple; try and find a ripe one

1 tablespoon of olive oil

1/4 teaspoon ground cloves

1 teaspoon cinnamon

2 tablespoons honey

1 tablespoon lime juice

Preparation Method

Mix the olive oil, cloves, honey, cinnamon and lime juice in a bowl. This will be used as the marinade.

Cut the leaves off of the pineapple.

Cut the skin off the pineapple in a vertical fashion.

Slice it in half lengthwise after it is bare.

Slice the core out of the pineapple slices.

Mix the pineapple with the marinade and grill for 3-4 minutes while basting the marinade on it once or twice.

Move the pineapple to a cooler part of your grill and baste the marinade on it again.

Grill the pineapple for three more minutes after adding the marinade.

The nutrient content of this meal is as follows:

Total Fat	2 g
Saturated Fat	0 g
Protein	0 g
Carbohydrate	15 g
Cholesterol	0 mg
Sodium	1 mg
Calories	79
Potassium	60 mg
Calcium	0 mg
Magnesium	50 mg
Fiber	1 g

Tuna Salad

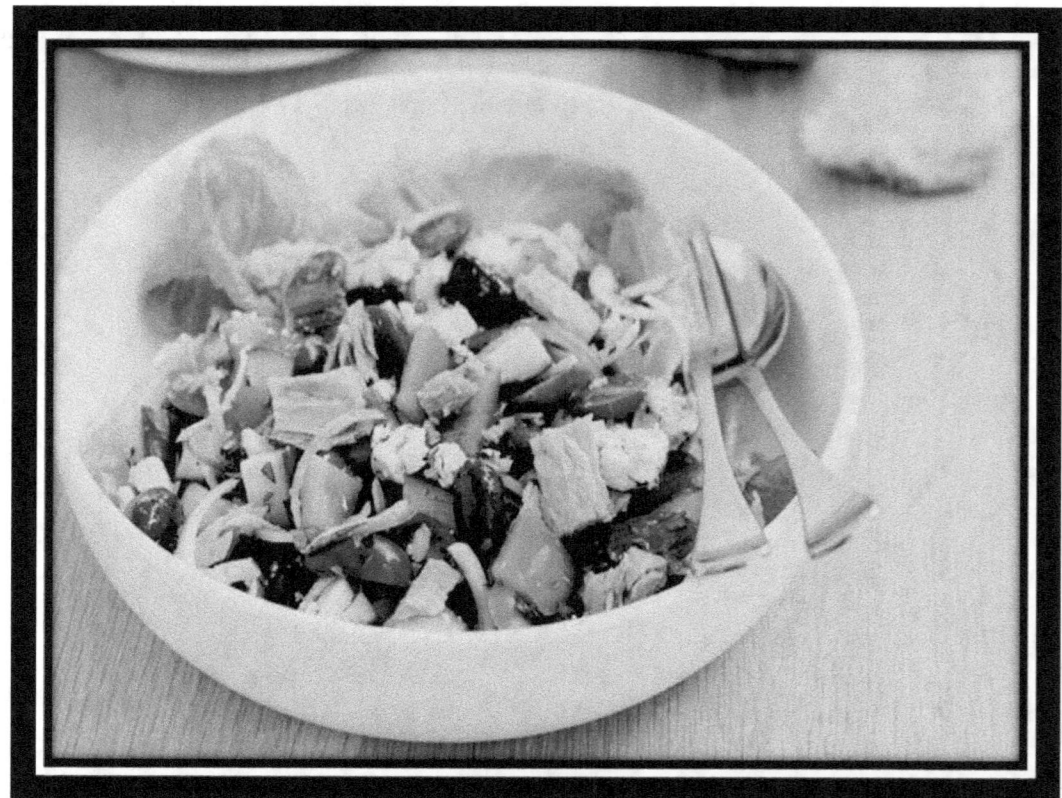

Serves 5 and requires 10 minutes to cook

Ingredients

6 tablespoons low fat mayonnaise

1/2 cup chopped green onions

2 cans water pack tuna

1/2 cup chopped raw celery

Preparation Method

Rinse the tuna and drain for 5 minutes.

Break the tuna to pieces with a fork.

Mix in the celery, mayonnaise and onions properly.

Serve.

The nutrient content of this meal is as follows:

Total Fat	7 g
Saturated Fat	1 g
Protein	16 g
Carbohydrate	2 g
Cholesterol	25 mg
Sodium	171 mg
Calories	138
Potassium	198 mg
Calcium	17 mg
Magnesium	19 mg
Fiber	0 g

Meatloaf Turkey

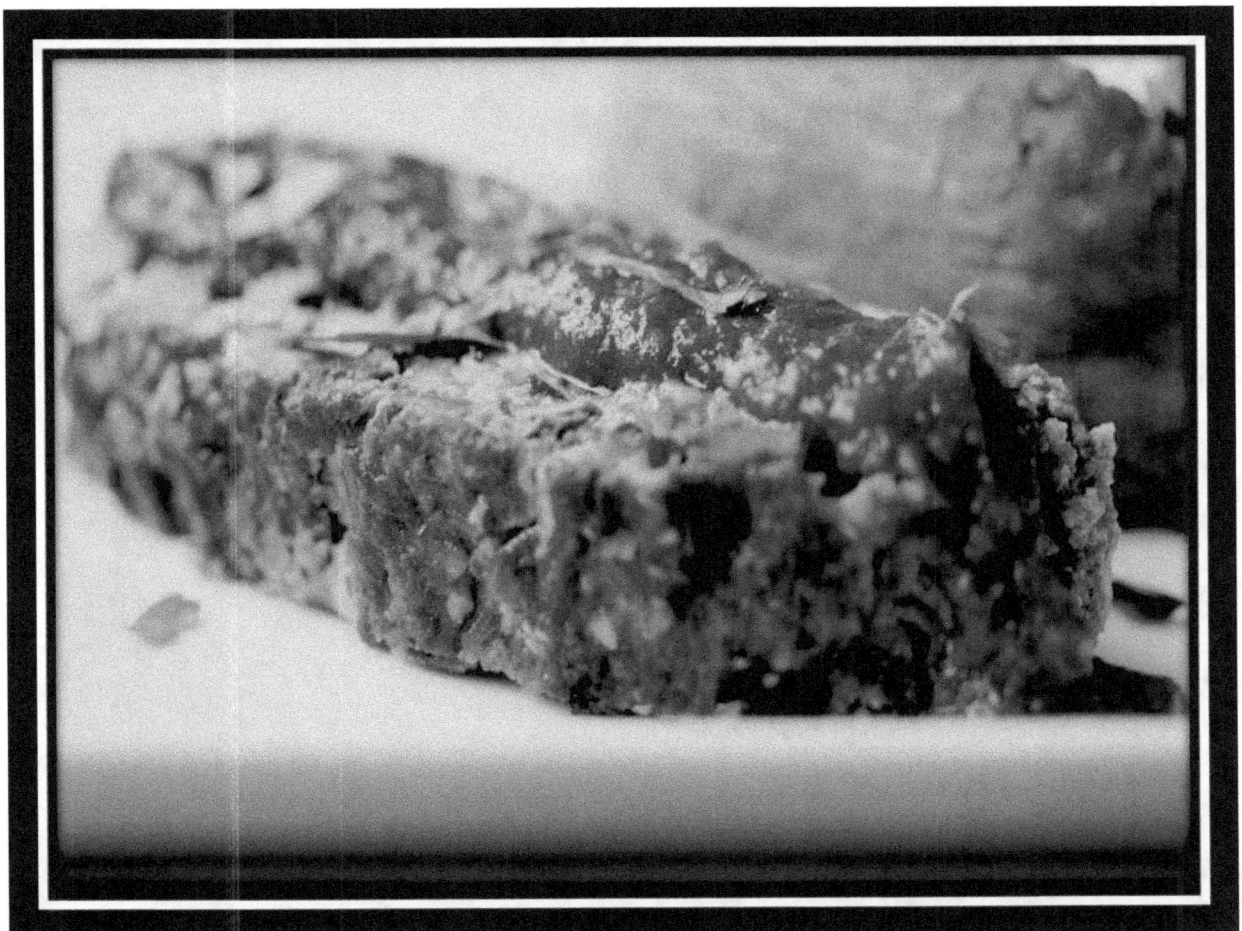

Serves 5, requires 35 minutes of time

Ingredients

1 pound ground turkey (lean)

1/4 cup low sodium ketchup

1 tablespoon dehydrated onion flakes

1 whole egg (large)

1/2 cup dry oats (regular)

Preparation Method

Set an oven to 350 degrees Fahrenheit.

Add all the ingredients together and mix well.

Use a low-fat material to lubricate the loaf pan.

Bake for 25 minutes inside the loaf pan.

Cut it into 5 slices and serve.

The nutrient content of this meal is as follows:

Total Fat	7 g
Saturated Fat	2 g
Protein	23 g
Carbohydrate	9 g
Cholesterol	103 mg
Sodium	205 mg
Calories	191
Potassium	268 mg
Calcium	24 mg
Magnesium	33 mg
Fiber	1 g

Whole Wheat Pretzel

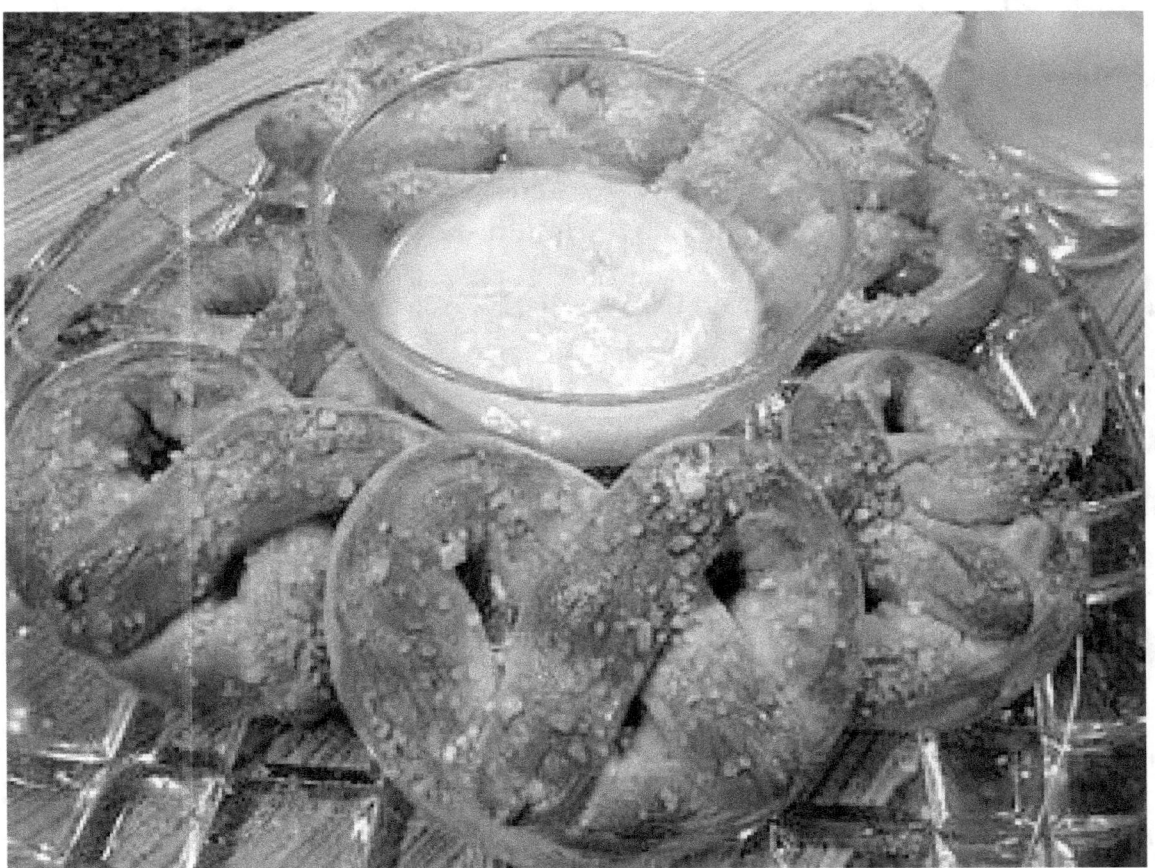

Serves 8, takes 30 minutes

Ingredients

1 package of active dry yeast

2 teaspoons of brown sugar

1/2 teaspoon salt

1 1/2 cups water

1 cup bread flour

3 cups whole-wheat flour

1/4 cup baking soda

1/2 cup of wheat gluten

1 tablespoon olive oil

Preparation Method

Mix the water, yeast, sugar and salt in a bowl for five minutes.

All the olive oil, gluten and flours after the five minutes are over.

Mix by hand for 10 minutes. The dough should start to form after a while.

Place the dough in a secure space with a plastic cover over it. Leave the cover on for an hour so the dough has time to rise.

Punch down the dough and roll it into eight pieces.

Roll each piece into a rope and make U shapes with them to create pretzel shapes or any other shape you want.

Boil 8-10 cups of water with the baking soda.

Add each pretzel on in an individual basis and cover for thirty seconds each, dipping them in the mixture.

Bake all the pretzels at 450 degrees Fahrenheit for 15 minutes.

Serve after the pretzels are nice and brown.

The nutrient content of this meal is as follows:

Total Fat	2 g
Saturated Fat	0 g
Protein	10 g
Carbohydrate	30 g
Cholesterol	0 mg
Sodium	105 mg
Calories	180
Potassium	0 mg
Calcium	0 mg
Magnesium	10 mg
Fiber	4 g

Salad Dressing, Yogurt

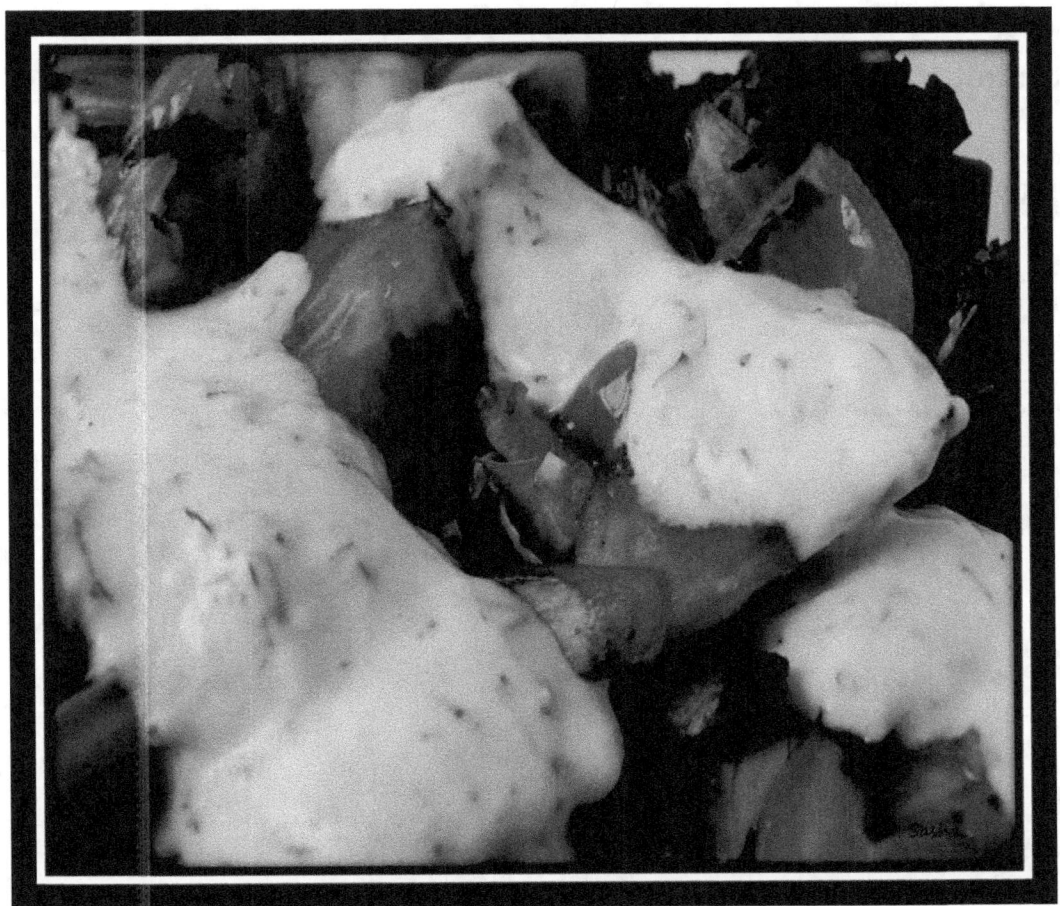

Serves 5, ready in 5 minutes

Ingredients

2 tablespoons lemon juice

2 tablespoons dried dill

2 tablespoons dried chives

8 oz. fat plain fat free yogurt

1/4 cup low fat mayonnaise

Preparation Method

Mix all the ingredients together in a bowl.

Store in a refrigerator and serve chilled.

The nutrient content of this meal is as follows:

Total Fat	2 g
Saturated Fat	0 g
Protein	2 g
Carbohydrate	4 g
Cholesterol	3 mg
Sodium	66 mg
Calories	39
Potassium	110 mg
Calcium	76 mg
Magnesium	10 mg
Fiber	0 g

Baked Fish (Spicy)

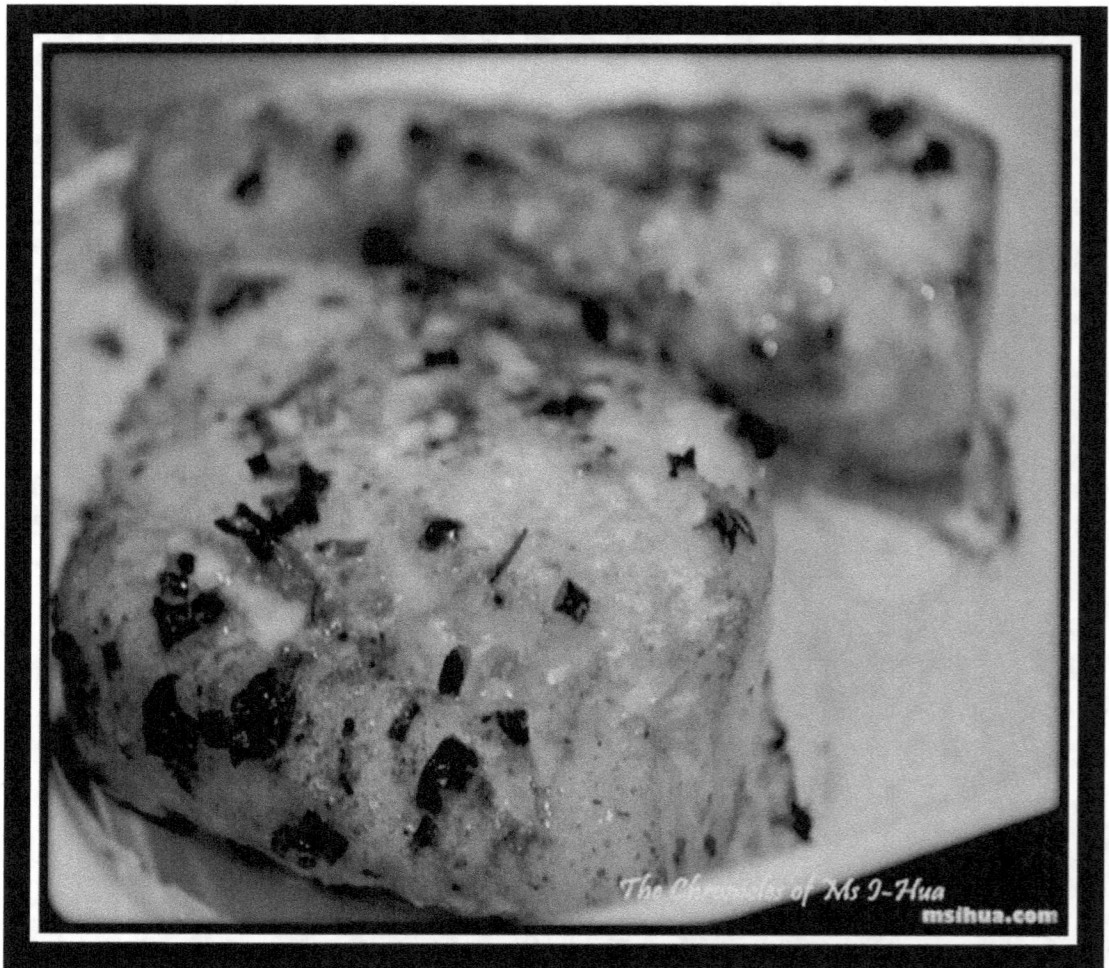

Serves 4, takes 25 minutes to prepare

Ingredients

1 teaspoon salt free spicy seasoning

1 pound salmon fillet or any other fish fillet

1 tablespoon olive oil

Preparation Method

Preheat the oven to 350 degrees Fahrenheit.

Spray some cooking oil on a casserole dish.

Wash the fish and dry properly, then put in a dish.

Mix together seasoning and oil then drizzle over the fish.

Bake for 15 minutes without covering.

Cut to 4 pieces and serve, particularly with rice.

The nutrient content of this meal is as follows:

Total Fat	11 g
Saturated Fat	2 g
Protein	23 g
Carbohydrate	Less than 1 g
Cholesterol	63 mg
Sodium	50 mg
Calories	192
Potassium	560 mg
Calcium	18 mg
Magnesium	34 mg
Fiber	0 g

Scallion Rice

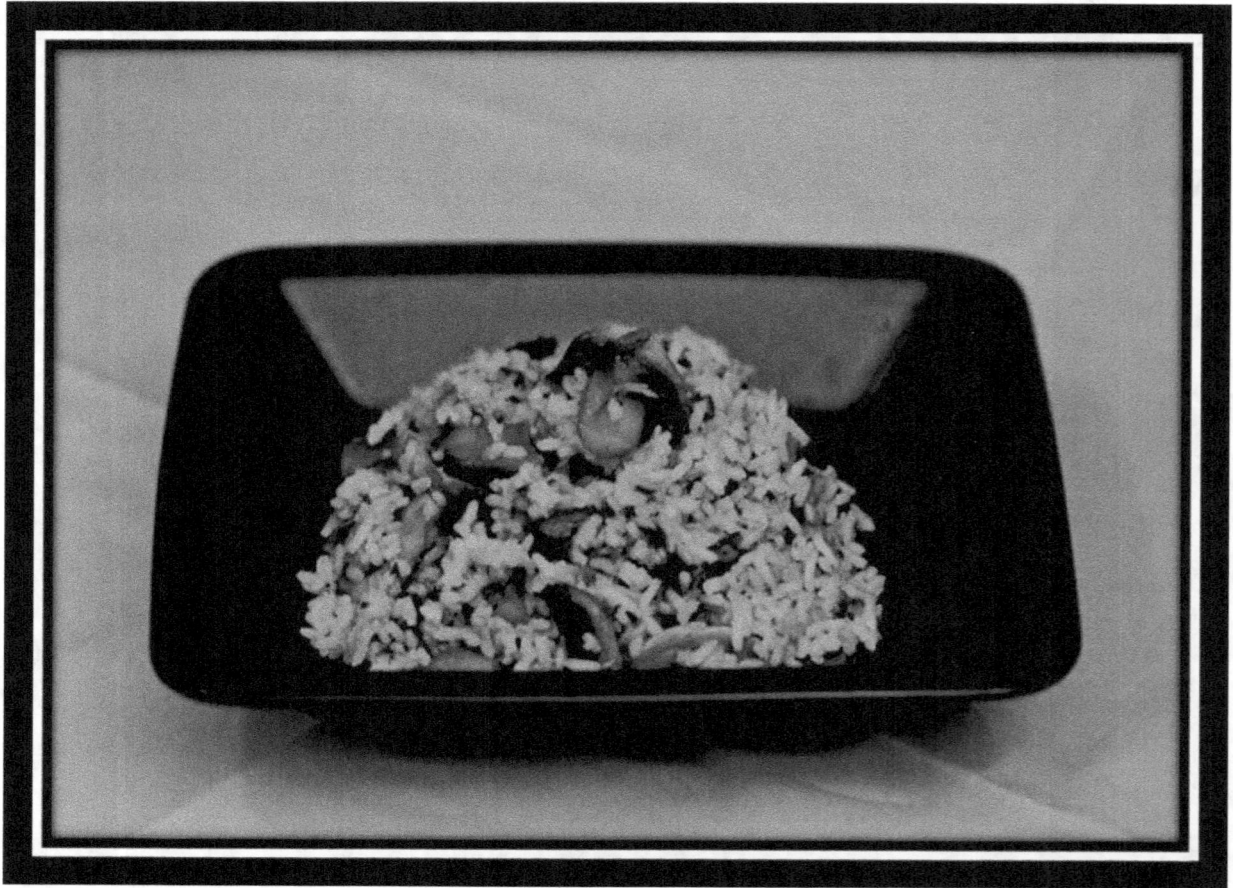

Serves 5 and takes 10 minutes to make

Ingredients

1/2 cup green chopped scallions

1 1/2 teaspoon low sodium bouillon granules

4 1/2 cups brown cooked rice (prepared in unsalted water)

Preparation Method

Take a bowl and combine the cooked rice (prepare according to the package standards) and the other ingredients together and then mix properly to serve.

The nutrient content of this meal is as follows:

Total Fat	2 g
Saturated Fat	0 g
Protein	5 g
Carbohydrate	41 g
Cholesterol	0 mg
Sodium	18 mg
Calories	200
Potassium	92 mg
Calcium	23 mg
Magnesium	77 mg
Fiber	6 g

Lasagna – Zucchini

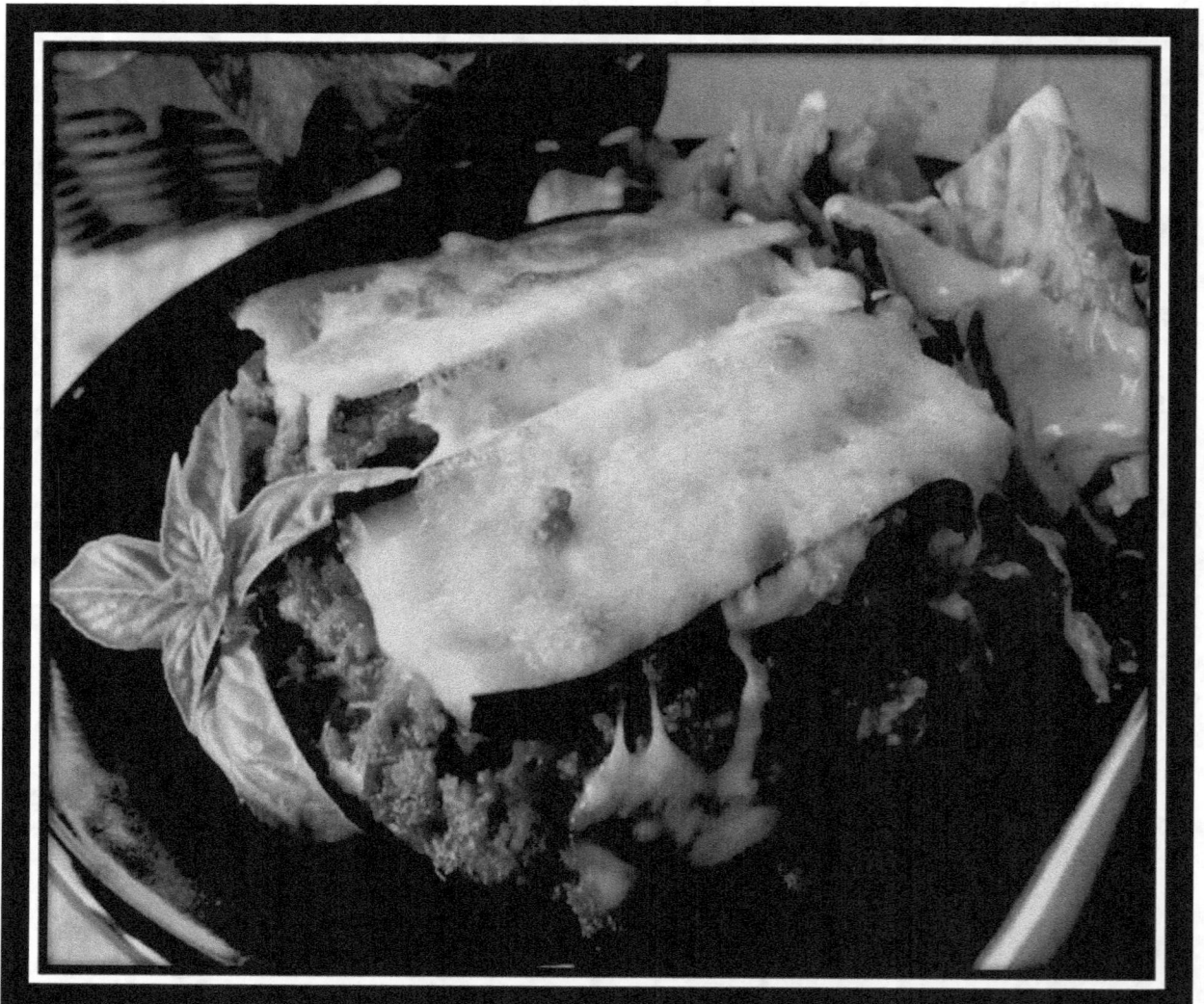

Serves 6, takes 1 hour to cook

Ingredients

1/8 teaspoon black pepper

1 garlic clove

1/4 cup chopped onions

2 teaspoons dried oregano

2 teaspoons dried basil

2 1/2 cups low sodium tomato sauce

1 1/2 cups raw sliced zucchini

1/4 cup grated parmesan cheese

1 1/2 cups fat free cottage cheese

3/4 cup grated part skimmed mozzarella cheese

1/2 pound cooked lasagna noodles (prepared with unsalted water)

Preparation Method

Bring an oven to heat at 350 degrees Fahrenheit.

Spray a baking dish with vegetable oil.

Mix together in a bowl 1/8 cup mozzarella and a tablespoon of parmesan cheese and let it rest.

Take another bowl and combine the remaining parmesan cheese and mozzarella cheese and then set it aside.

Take another bowl and mix tomato sauce and all of the other ingredients.

Layer the tomato sauce at the bottom of the baking dish.

Add another layer of noodles (about 1/3 of the noodles).

Spread 1/2 of the cheese mixture on it then put a layer of zucchini.

Repeat the layers again then set a sauce coating on the rest of the noodles; this should incorporate the sauce and cheese mixture that you set aside earlier.

Cover with aluminum foil.

Bake for 35 - 40 minutes.

Allow to cool for 15 – 20 minutes.

Cut to six portions and serve.

The nutrient content of this meal is as follows:

Total Fat	5 g
Saturated Fat	3 g
Protein	15 g
Carbohydrate	24 g
Cholesterol	12 mg
Sodium	368 mg
Calories	200
Potassium	593 mg
Calcium	310 mg
Magnesium	46 mg
Fiber	3 g

Fruit & Nut Bar

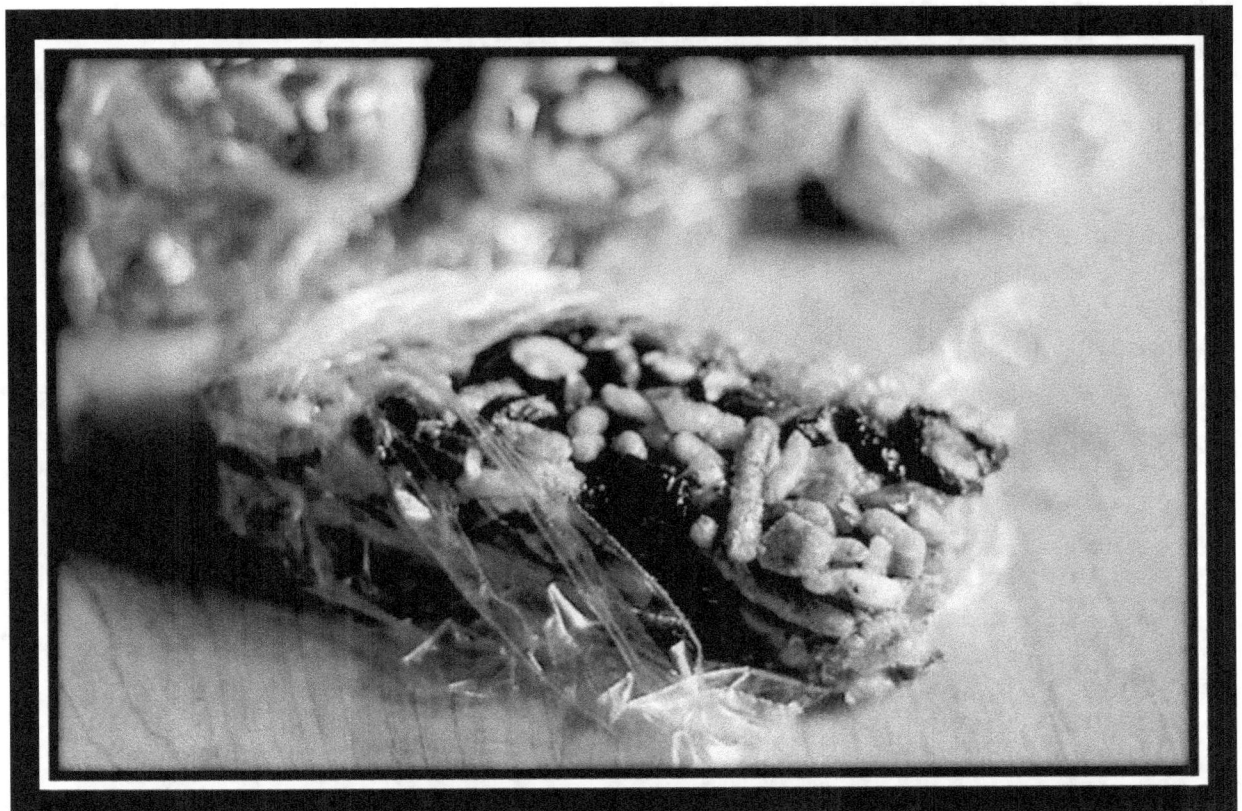

This meal should prepare enough for 10 people and takes 30 minutes

Ingredients

1/2 cup quinoa flour

2 tablespoons corn starch

1/4 cup dried pineapple, chopped

1/2 cup oats

1/4 cup buckwheat honey

1/4 cup dried figs, chopped

1/4 cup flax meal

1/4 cup almonds, chopped

1/4 cup wheat germ

1/4 cup dried apricots

Preparation Method

Take all the ingredients together and mix them properly.

Take a parchment lined sheet pan and spread half an inch thick of the mixture.

Bake for 20 minutes at 300 degrees Fahrenheit.

Cool and cut so you can serve.

The nutrient content of this meal is as follows:

Total Fat	1 g
Saturated Fat	Negligible
Protein	2 g
Calories	61
Carbohydrate	11 g
Cholesterol	0 mg
Sodium	5 mg
Sugars	7 g
Trans fat	0 mg
Monounsaturated fat	0.5 mg
Fiber	1 g

Green Smoothie

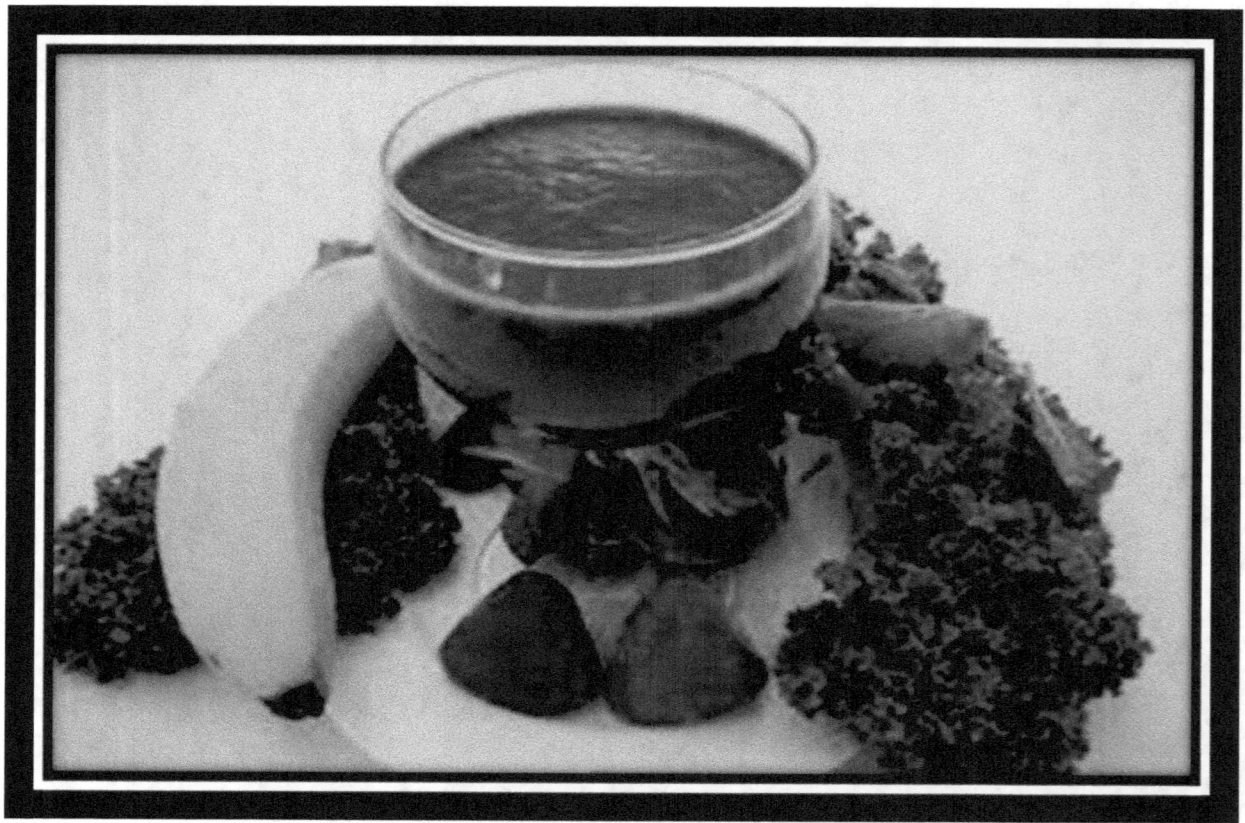

This meal serves 4 and can be ready in just 5 minutes

Ingredients

Cold water or ice (1 cup)

1 banana

1 tablespoon fresh mint

1/2 cup strawberries

2 ounces fresh baby spinach

4 tablespoons Lemon juice

1/2 cup other kinds of berries

Preparation Method

Put all the ingredients in a blender or a juicer and mix properly.

Serve after everything is blended; try to serve chilled if possible.

The nutrient content of this meal is as follows:

Total Fat	Negligible
Saturated Fat	Negligible
Protein	1 g
Calories	52
Carbohydrate	12 g
Cholesterol	0 mg
Sodium	14 mg
Sugars	0 g
Trans fat	0 mg
Monounsaturated fat	Negligible
Fiber	2 g

Island Chiller

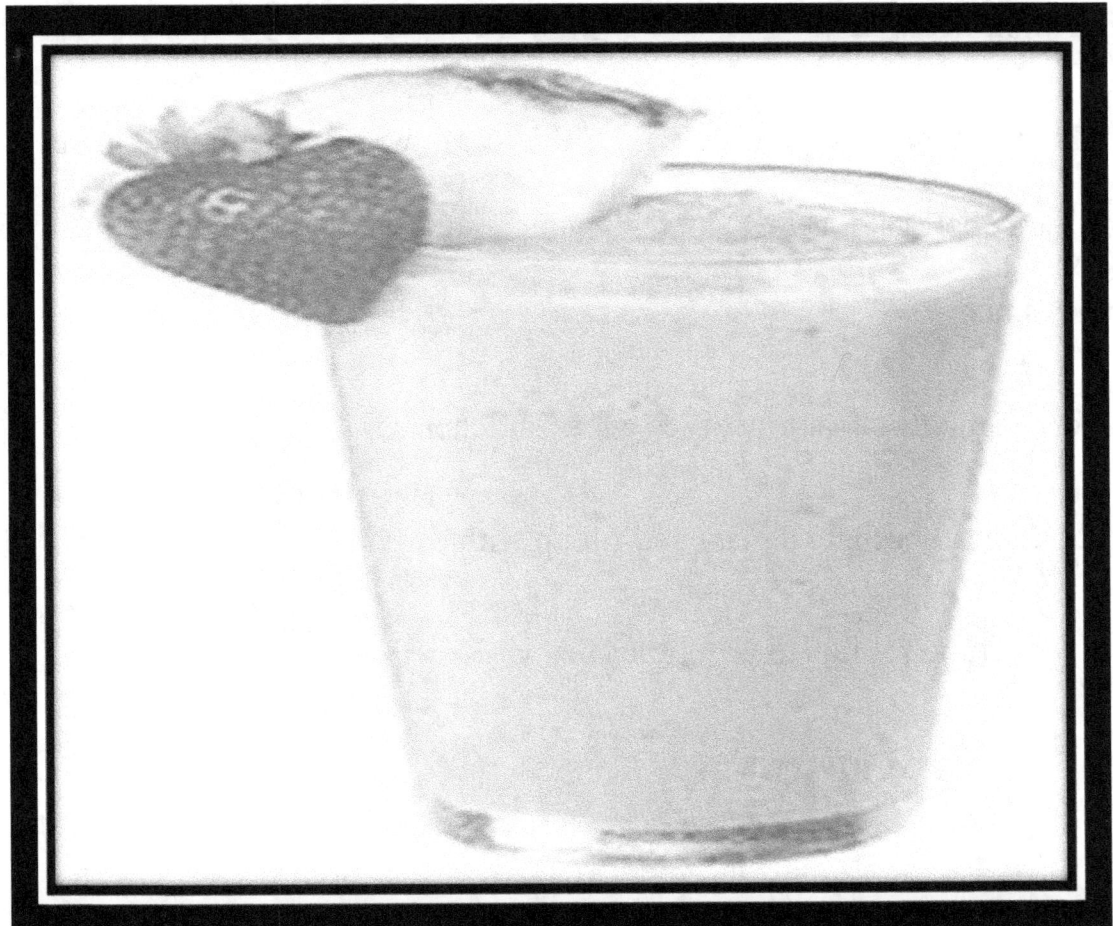

This is good for 16 servings

Ingredients

2 packages of unsweetened strawberries

16 fresh strawberries

Chilled carbonated water, 2 quarts

3 cups orange juice

Crushed pineapple with the juice, 1 can

Preparation Method

Take the pineapple, the pineapple juice that came with it, the orange juice and the frozen strawberries together in a blender and mix properly until the mixture becomes smooth.

Transfer the mixture to a tray of ice cubes and then set it in the freezer.

Take 2 – 3 ice cubes into a glass and fill up with carbonated water to taste.

Allow some time for this to be a little slushy.

Garnish with strawberries and serve.

The nutrient content of this meal is as follows:

Total Fat	0 g
Saturated Fat	0 g
Protein	1 g
Calories	68
Carbohydrate	16 g
Cholesterol	0 mg
Sodium	6 mg
Monounsaturated fat	0 mg
Fiber	1 g

Conclusion

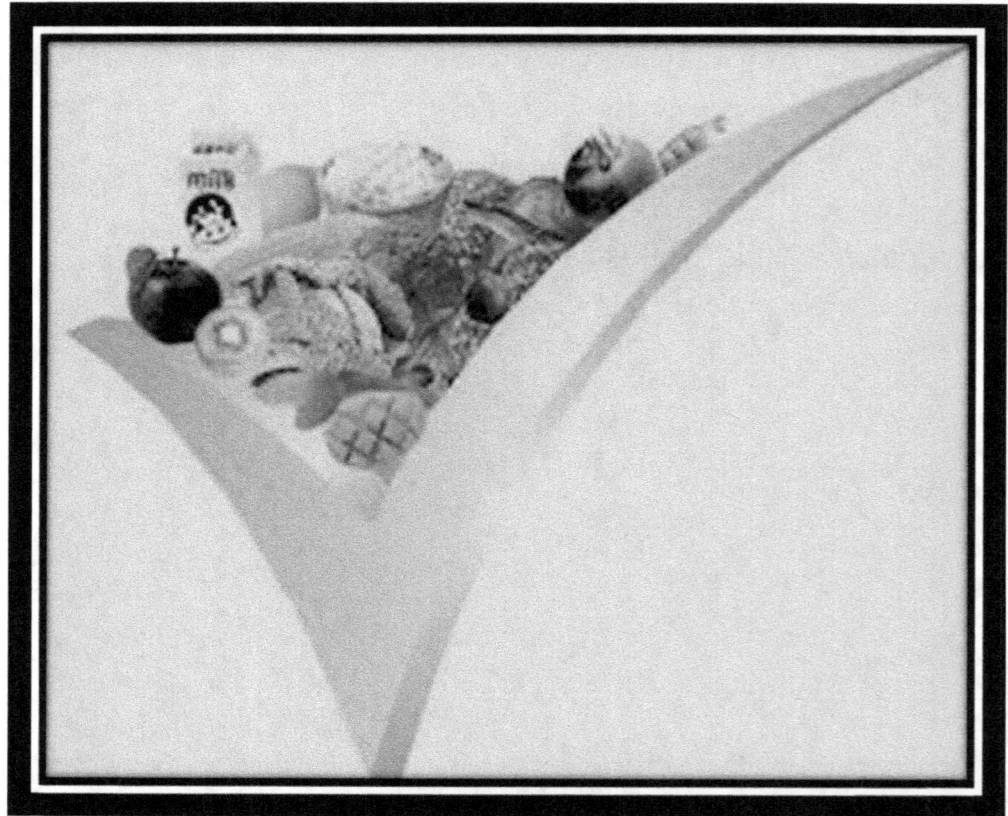

When it comes to the issue of staying healthy, it is important that we watch what we eat. This is of course in the face of the fact that a lot of the foods that we eat today contribute to a large extent to the diseases and illnesses that we suffer.

Blood pressure is not something that we should take for granted, and as a matter of fact it is important for us to make sure that we have our blood pressure in check. In the event that you realize that your blood pressure is not according to what is considered the optimal level, it is important for you to try and seek medical advice as soon as possible.

The DASH Diet is one of the best alternatives that can help you overcome hypertension and other related issues. It really is not a very hard diet to be on as compared to most of the other diets that are available in the market today. There are several sources of information from which you can learn as much as you can about the diet, and it is from such that you should be able to get more information about the diet and the foods that it utilizes.

From this book, you should have learned the basics of the DASH Diet and all you will ever need to know if you wish to start on the plan. Remember that this book is usable by both beginners and novices to the DASH Diet, and as long as you follow the guidelines carefully, it will be very easy for you to ensure a good state of health.

There are a number of recipes that have also been included in the book to give you a rough idea of what to make just in case you do not have an idea of how to go about meals on this diet. Apart from the diet recipes, there are also a number of foods that have been listed from which you can also consume. Therefore, you should be in a good position to set out on a DASH Diet and reap the benefits that come with it.

It is my hope when writing this book that your life will be enhanced through the work I have done, and most importantly that you will find this book useful in keeping you and your family in a sound state of health.

All the Best!